Handbook of
LASIK SURGERY

Handbook of
LASIK SURGERY

RASIK B VAJPAYEE MBBS,MS
Professor of Ophthalmology
Director, Cornea Service
Dr Rajendra Prasad Centre for Ophthalmic Sciences
All India Institute of Medical Sciences
New Delhi

TANUJ DADA MD
Senior Registrar, Cornea Service
Dr Rajendra Prasad Centre for Ophthalmic Sciences
All India Institute of Medical Sciences
New Delhi

GRANT R SNIBSON FRACS, FRACO, FRCOphth
Senior Lecturer, University of Melbourne
Department of Ophthalmology
Senior Specialist
Royal Victorian Eye and Ear Hospital, Melbourne
Member, Melbourne Excimer Laser Group

HUGH R TAYLOR MD, FRACS, FRACO, FACS
Ringland Anderson Professor, University of Melbourne
Department of Ophthalmology
Head Corneal Unit, Royal Victorian Eye and Ear Hospital, Melbourne
Scientific Director, Melbourne Excimer Laser Group

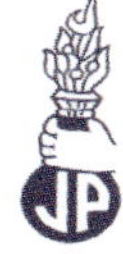

JAYPEE BROTHERS
MEDICAL PUBLISHERS (P) LTD
New Delhi

Published by

Jitendar P Vij
Jaypee Brothers Medical Publishers (P) Ltd
B-3 EMCA House, 23/23B Ansari Road, Daryaganj
Post Box 7193, New Delhi 110 002, India
Phones: 3272143, 3272703, 3282021   Fax: 011-3276490
E-mail: jpmedpub@del2.vsnl.net.in
Visit our web site: http://www.clinichem.com

Branches

- 202 Batavia Chambers, 8 Kumara Kruppa Road
  Kumara Park East, **Bangalore** 560 001
  Phone: 2285971, 2281761 (Tele Fax)
  E-mail: jaypeebc@bgl.vsnl.net.in
- 1A Indian Mirror Street, Wellington Square
  Calcutta 700 013, Phone: 2451926 Fax: 2456075
  E-mail: jpbcal@cal.vsnl.net.in
- 282 IIIrd Floor, Khaleel Shirazi Estate, Fountain Plaza
  Pantheon Road, **Chennai** 600 008, Phone: 8262665 Fax: 8262331
  E-mail: jpmedpub@md3.vsnl.net.in
- 106 Amit Industrial Estate, 61 Dr SS Rao Road
  Near MGM Hospital, Parel, **Mumbai** 400 012
  Phone: 4124863 Fax: 4160828
  E-mail: jpmedpub@bom7.vsnl.net.in

Handbook of LASIK Surgery

This book has been published on good faith and belief that the material provided by authors is original. Every effort is made to ensure accuracy of material, but the publisher, printer and authors will not be held responsible for any inadvertent error(s). In case of any dispute, all legal matters to be settled under Delhi jurisdiction only.

First Edition : 2000

ISBN 81-7179-726-1

Typeset at   JPBMP typesetting unit
Printed at   Lordson Publishers (P) Ltd., C-5/19, Rana Pratap Bagh, Delhi 110 007

to
my parents
Late Kamla and Avadh Vajpayee

—Rasik B Vajpayee

to
my parents for their unconditional
love and for nurturing me into a
compassionate clinician

—Tanuj Dada

to
my wife Pam
and
children Kaela and Nikita

—Grant R Snibson

to
my wife Liz

—Hugh R Taylor

Foreword

Inevitably, spheres of human endeavours start simply and become more complex. This principle is well illustrated by refractive surgery. In 1980, only two techniques of refractive surgery were practised worldwide: refractive keratotomy for myopia and astigmatism and cryolathe keratomileusis. Now, 20 years later, approximately 20 different refractive surgical techniques — some obsolete, many in routine use, and an increasing number in active new development — vie for the attention of ophthalmic surgeons and raise the hopes of ametropic patients. Laser *in-situ* keratomileusis (LASIK) is currently the most widely used of these techniques.

The problem is, LASIK itself has become extremely complex. The procedure is a fusion of keratomileusis (which had its roots in the cryolathe techniques of Barraquer and the *in-situ* techniques of Ruiz) and excimer laser photoablation (which had its roots in microchip manufacturing and was brought to refractive surgery by Trokel and Srinivasan) — a fusion formulated by Pallikaris — LASIK's many physical, technical, biological, and clinical facets dazzle the ophthalmic surgeon — particularly a beginner.

By parallel, when refractive keratotomy was in common use, the surgeons confronted with hundreds of peer-reviewed articles, endless newspaper columns and a "classic" 1300-page textbook understandably shrunk from the task of interpreting and absorbing this mammoth amount of information, so shorter handbook style publications became available.

Current LASIK textbooks span hundred of pages and the periodical literature hundreds of articles. Where can the students, the surgeons, and the practitioners who seek a concise presentation of LASIK turn? The answer is in your hands — this *Handbook*. This superb, concise volume contains the essential information to orient a beginning surgeon who plans to operate on and manage patients with LASIK. It can serve as a meaningful review for the active refractive surgeons as well as optometrists and others who want access to the basic information. Outlining the principles of photoablation, the important facets of patient selection for surgery, the features of different models of microkeratomes and excimer lasers, surgical techniques, and the recognition and management of complications, the authors have served readers well by assembling the basics in one useful volume.

In such a fast moving field, there are observations in the book that become outdated by the time they are read and newer information that is not yet included. Such small difficulties detract minimally from the beauty of this highly practical and useful volume.

George O Waring III
MD FACS FRCOphth
Professor of Ophthalmology
Emory University School of Medicine
Atlanta, Georgia

Preface

The last decade has seen a technological explosion in the field of excimer laser surgery. Currently laser-in-situ keratomileusis (LASIK) is the most popular refractive procedure among ophthalmologists and patients alike. The volume of literature on this subject is enormous and ever-expanding. Although a number of textbooks are available on LASIK, to date there are very few single source documents that provide practical reference information.

With these facts in mind we have endeavoured to create a practical, well-illustrated and user-friendly handbook emphasising the salient features of LASIK surgery. The handbook provides reader with the basic knowledge about excimer laser technology, the various microkeratomes used for creation of the corneal flap and gives detailed information about the preoperative assessment, the surgical technique and the prevention and management of the complications associated with LASIK. In addition we have given information on a repeat LASIK procedure and LASIK done for residual errors after previous surgical procedures, such as radial keratotomy and penetrating keratoplasty. A review of the results of LASIK in myopia, hyperopia and astigmatism is also included.

This handbook aims at providing useful information for practicing ophthalmologists and can be consulted by refractive surgeons to solve frequently encountered problems related to the evaluation, treatment and postoperative management of patients undergoing LASIK.

Rasik B Vajpayee
Tanuj Dada
Grant R Snibson
Hugh R Taylor

Acknowledgements

We wish to express our heartfelt gratitude to Prof VK Dada, Chief of Dr Rajendra Prasad Centre for Ophthalmic Sciences, All India Institute of Medical Sciences, New Delhi, who has been a source of constant inspiration and guidance. We would also like to thank Dr Namrata Sharma, Suman, Sudha, Anu and Vikas for their assistance in the preparation of the manuscript.

Contents

One

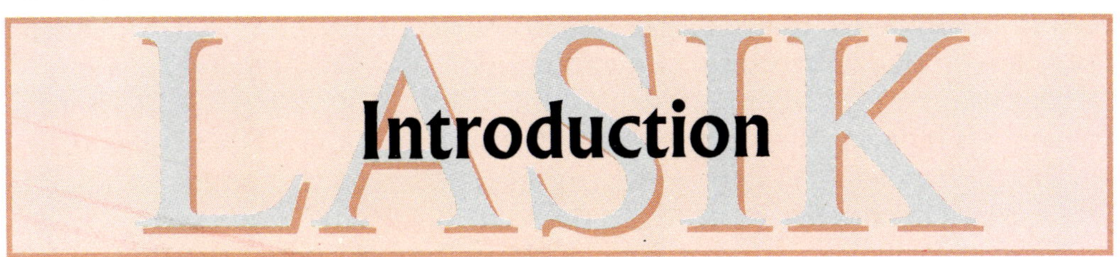

INTRODUCTION

Mankind has strived for excellence in every sphere of life including the medical sciences. Not only have there been miraculous innovations to cure several of the diseases that afflict our race, rapid strides have also been made in the medical field to cure the naturally occurring defects in the human body. Refractive error is one such defect that affects millions of people worldwide.

External aids such as spectacles and contact lenses have been used to treat the various refractive errors. However these aids have several drawbacks. Spectacles significantly modify the size of the retinal image, reduce the field of vision, cannot be used for high degrees of anisometropia, are cosmetically unacceptable to many people and are job hazards in various occupations. Contact lenses take care of many of these problems, but require meticulous cleaning, daily wear and removal, induce allergic reactions, increase the risk of infection and may not be tolerated by many patients. In the past few years, the technique of refractive surgery has evolved and gained wide acceptance in the public. This has been possible due to an improved knowledge of the anatomy and physiology of the eye and the explosive developments in technology. Fyodorov's radial keratotomy (RK), a popular procedure in the last decade has fallen into disrepute due to its relative unpredictability, inability to treat high refractive errors, a permanent structural weakening of the cornea and various associated complications. Trokel and Srinivasan introduced photorefractive keratectomy (PRK) which revolutionised the field of refractive surgery and is still a popular procedure in many parts of the world. However the limelight has now been shifted to the new refractive procedure of laser-*in-situ* keratomileusis (LASIK).

PRINCIPLE OF THE EXCIMER LASER

The excimer laser is a high-energy ultraviolet laser used to ablate corneal tissues at a predictable rate. The word *excimer* is derived from *excited dimer* which stands for an energised molecule with two identical components. Actually the excimer laser is composed of a gas mixture with two different molecules. The mixture is composed of a rare gas (argon, xenon or krypton) and a halogen (fluoride, chloride or bromide). Argon fluoride is the most common gas used. The application of a high-voltage current (approx. 30,000 eV) leads to the formation of highly unstable rare gas halide molecules, which rapidly dissociate emitting ultraviolet (UV) light with a wavelength dependent on the particular gas mixture (193 nm in case of Argon fluoride).

The far UV photons thus emitted, break up the intramolecular bonds with minimal thermal damage to the surrounding structures, a process known as *ablative photodecomposition or photoablation*. The laser is first absorbed by the tissues and results in intramolecular bond breakage. Subsequently, there is a large increase in the volume of the decomposed tissue and the kinetic energy of the photons ejects this decomposed tissue out of the surgical plane. With an energy density (energy per unit area or fluence) ranging between 50 and 300 mJ/cm^2, the excimer laser is capable of precise removal of corneal tissues. Each laser pulse ablates a tissue layer that is 0.25 µm thick and converts it into a gaseous material.

PRK *vs.* LASIK

Laser-*in-situ* keratomileusis (LASIK) is the latest technique of excimer laser refractive surgery, that is currently being used by refractive surgeons for the correction of various types of refractive errors. For many corneal surgeons, LASIK has become the technique of choice to correct moderate and high degrees of myopia, with or without astigmatism and for hypermetropia. LASIK is a modification of excimer laser photorefractive keratectomy [PRK], in which the excimer laser is used to ablate superficial corneal stromal tissue after the epithelium has been removed. LASIK involves the use of a microkeratome to prepare a hinged corneal flap of uniform thickness. The excimer laser is subsequently used to ablate the mid-corneal stromal bed and the flap is thereafter reposited to its original place without any sutures. After LASIK, the healing of corneal tissue occurs quickly since there is minimal damage to the corneal epithelium and the Bowman's layer.

The advantages of LASIK over surface PRK relate to a number of factors. PRK requires a large area of de-epithelialisation and the removal of the Bowman's layer. This leads to the formation of a new epithelial layer which is often hyper-plastic, disorganisation of the stromal collagen fibres, and the deposition of new collagen fibres below the epithelial layer. In contrast, removal of the epithelium is not required in LASIK, there are minimal postoperative epithelial alterations, the integrity of the Bowman's membrane is maintained, there is a greater respect to stromal fibre organisation and a reduced histological response. These factors translate into rapid healing and increased postoperative patient comfort, minimal corneal haze, early stability with little regression, faster visual rehabilitation and minimal need if any for steroid therapy. However, a major disadvantage of LASIK is its dependence on the creation of the corneal flap with a microkeratome, a procedure that has its own set of potential complications.

The microkeratomes are expensive and delicate instruments that require meticulous handling and maintenance. Although rapid strides are being made in microkeratome technology, the currently available instruments which use a steel or diamond blade or a water jet to cut across the corneal stroma, are far from perfect. The introduction of laser keratomes in the near future may overcome this handicap. Furthermore problems can arise from the flap itself. These include irregularity, malposition or displacement of the flap, occurrence of irregular astigmatism and ingrowth of corneal epithelium beneath the flap. With improvement in the designs of the microkeratomes and in the surgical protocols, the incidence of flap-related complications is being reduced, and most studies of LASIK now report quite impressive results. The technique of LASIK has become an integral part of refractive surgery and is currently regarded as the preferred surgical technique for the correction of a large spectrum of refractive errors.

Two

History and Development

The history of modern refractive surgery dates back to 1949 when Jose I Barraquer proposed the surgical modification of the refractive status of the eye by changing the radius of curvature of the anterior corneal surface. Initially, Barraquer experimented on performing a free hand lamellar dissection of the corneal stroma to create a lamellar corneal disc and then attempted a refractive cut by removing stromal tissue from the bed (keratomileusis-*in-situ*) or the stromal surface of the corneal disc. He then considered freezing the lamellar corneal disc and used the cryolathe to modify its profile. In 1958, Barraquer performed the first such procedure in a human using a prototype keratome with cutting angle of zero degrees.

In the late 1980s, Luis Ruiz developed an automated microkeratome and reported that the refractive effect of stromal resection can be altered by varying its diameter and depth. The development of this microkeratome was a major advancement in the field of lamellar refractive surgery and the surgery came to be known as automated lamellar keratoplasty [ALK]. This microkeratome rendered a much smoother stromal bed due to the controlled speed of the advancement of the keratome head and the very high speed of oscillation of the blade. However, ALK had inherent complications such as lost or displaced caps, irregular astigmatism and was not a very predictable procedure. Furthermore the technique of ALK had a long learning curve and required considerable surgical skill and experience. With the development of the excimer laser technology, ALK became less popular.

Trokel and Srinivasan in 1983 suggested the first corneal application of the excimer laser and in 1988 the first surgical applications in normal sighted human eyes were performed by McDonald and Kaufman (PRK—photorefractive keratectomy).

In 1989, Lucio Buratto presented the technique of intrastromal keratomileusis using the excimer laser. He performed the refractive cut followed by laser ablation of the free lamellar corneal disc in combination with an *in-situ* ablation of the exposed stromal bed.

LASIK: IMPORTANT MILESTONES		
1958	Keratomileusis	Barraquer
1962	Manual Microkeratome	Barraquer
1983	Corneal application of Excimer laser	Trokel and Srinivasan
1988	First successful PRK	McDonald
1989	Automated Microkeratome and ALK	Ruiz
1989	LASIK in normal human eye	Buratto
1990	Hinge technique in LASIK	Pallikaris
1991	Sutureless LASIK	Avalos,Guimaraes

Pallikaris and his colleagues in 1990, made the next major advancement in the field of LASIK surgery when they introduced the *hinge technique* for LASIK, by using a flap with a nasal hinge instead of a free flap.

In 1991, Avalos and Guimaraes described a sutureless LASIK technique, while Buratto in 1996 started using a Hansatome that made a vertical cut and a superior hinge. Since then a number of improvements have taken place in excimer laser delivery and microkeratomes, and the current literature bears testimony to the fact that LASIK has developed into a relatively safe and effective refractive procedure.

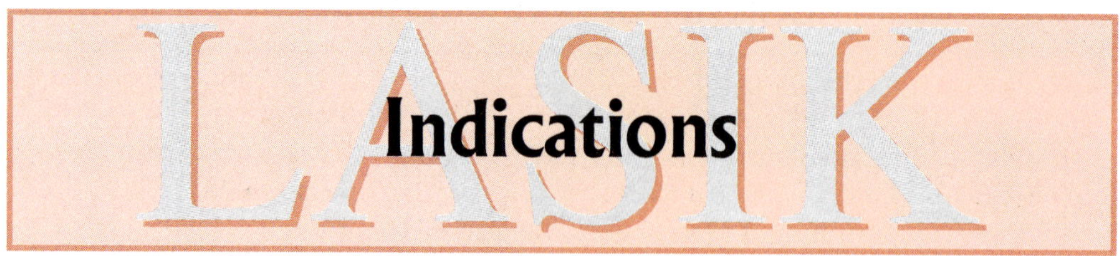

Three

Indications

Laser-in-situ keratomileusis (LASIK) was initially used to correct higher magnitudes of myopia and many refractive surgeons found it to be superior to photorefractive keratectomy (PRK). Subsequently due to the various advantages of LASIK, such as a reduced patient discomfort, rapid healing, early visual rehabilitation, minimal corneal haze and better predictability, the utility of the procedure was expanded for the correction of many forms of refractive errors. Currently LASIK is being used to treat the following.

Myopia

Laser-in-situ keratomileusis (LASIK) has been used to treat myopia ranging from –1 to –30 dioptres. However the correction of myopia of more than – 15 D entails excessive stromal ablation with a danger of producing the serious complication of corneal ectasia. The accuracy of the procedure and the patient satisfaction are also quite poor in myopia of more than –15 D. Therefore LASIK should be restricted to treat myopia of 15 D or less, while a phakic anterior chamber IOL or a clear-lens extraction with a negative power IOL, may be a better option for myopia of more than 15 D. It is important to remember that the amount of myopic correction possible in a particular patient is determined by the central corneal pachymetry and correction of myopic refractive errors in excess of 10 dioptres may not be possible if the central pachymetry is less than 500 µm.

Hypermetropia

Although the treatment of hyperopic refractive errors with LASIK started much later, LASIK can now be used to correct hypermetropia ranging from +1 to +8 dioptres. Although hyperopic LASIK appears to be a safe and effective procedure, there is a need for modification of the current algorithms and a better ablation profile to improve the predictability and the long term stability of this procedure.

Astigmatism

It has now become possible to treat myopic and hyperopic astigmatism with LASIK. Correction has been attempted in astigmatic errors ranging from –0.5 to

10 D, although the technique of astigmatic ablation is still being refined. In eyes with a mixed astigmatism it may not be possible to correct the entire error in a single ablation, and it is better to separate the refractive error into 2 components. For example, consider a refractive error, of – 2 D sph/+ 4 D cyl 180. Separate out half the cylinder (+ 2 cyl 180) such that the sphere and the cylinder are equal in magnitude but opposite in sign. Therefore the two components are (I) + 2 D cyl at 180 and (II) – 2 D sph/+2 D cyl 180. Now transpose (II) to get – 2 D cyl 90. This is the first laser treatment, while the remaining cylinder (+ 2 cyl 180), i.e. component (I), constitutes the second laser treatment.

Residual Refractive Errors after Previous Surgical Procedures

Laser-in-situ keratomileusis (LASIK) has been used to treat residual refractive errors after radial keratotomy, penetrating keratoplasty, epikeratoplasty and cataract surgery. Although the nomograms for LASIK after these procedures are still under development, impressive surgical results have been reported by various authors. It is vital to ensure adequate wound healing and rule out corneal thinning prior to considering LASIK surgery in these patients.

Four

Preoperative Assessment

PATIENT SELECTION

The patient selection in any refractive procedure is of vital importance. Preoperative patient education and a thorough understanding of the risks and benefits involved in the surgery are essential. The patient should have a practical knowledge of the procedure which can be obtained from brochures, video presentations and by consultation with the surgeon.

All potential complications and limitations of the procedure should be discussed with the patient. In patients nearing the presbyopic age group, the need for reading glasses after the surgery must be clearly explained. The patients should be made to understand that the procedure may have to be aborted intraoperatively due to microkeratome or laser malfunction or if the surgical conditions are not ideal. Informed consent must be obtained prior to surgery.

Usually a patient is selected to undergo LASIK on the basis of both medical and personal requirements. Indications for LASIK to correct a refractive error include intolerance or refusal to wear contact lenses or spectacles and a desire of the patient to benefit from the refractive surgery. The refractive error of a candidate for the LASIK procedure should be stable for at least 12 months. Presence of ectasia or any other active corneal pathology and a corneal thickness of less than 450 μm is an absolute contraindication for LASIK. Dry eye, glaucoma, small palpebral aperture, sunken eye, monocular patient, a pupil size larger than the optic zone for the laser ablation, autoimmune disease, systemic or ocular vascular disease and pregnancy are some of the other relative contraindications for LASIK.

HISTORY

Stability of Refraction

It is important to make sure that the refractive error of a LASIK candidate is stable, at least for the preceding year. The results of refractive surgery in an eye

PATIENT SELECTION CRITERIA

1. Above 18 years of age
2. Stable refraction for at least 12 months
3. Refusal to wear glasses or contact lenses
4. Intolerance to contact lenses
5. Absence of corneal pathology
6. Realistic expectations from the procedure
7. Properly obtained informed consent

with a changing refractive error will be disappointing. LASIK is usually performed in patients who are 18 years or older, as at this age the refractive status of the eye has often stabilised and informed consent can be given. An indication of the stability of the patient's refraction can be obtained from the history of his or her earlier refractive status and assessment of the dioptric power of previous and current spectacles or contact lenses. The change in spherical equivalent should not be more than 0.50 dioptre over 12 months.

Contact Lens Wear

Contact lens wear can cause reversible changes in the refractive status of an eye due to its effect on the corneal curvature. Therefore, contact lens wearers are advised to discontinue the use of their lenses (*for at least one week in the case of soft lens users and four weeks in case of hard/RGP (rigid gas permeable) lens users)* prior to the preoperative evaluation and surgery. In the case of hard/ RGP lens users, if there is a change in the initial refraction of more than 0.5 D during the check-up at 4 weeks, the refractive status should be reassessed after 8 weeks or until the refraction is found to be stable. Sometimes corneal warpage occurs because of contact lens wear. In such a case, the preoperative evaluation may need to be deferred for some months after the patient has discontinued the use of contact lenses.

Medical and Ophthalmic Problems

The suitability of a candidate for LASIK surgery may be affected by a number of ocular and systemic problems. The following conditions should be ruled out as they can increase the risk for complications or an unsatisfactory outcome after LASIK. These may include lid problems (blepharitis), poor corrected visual acuity, active corneal or ocular surface disease, thin corneas, steep corneas, central corneal vascularisation, large pupil size, uncontrolled glaucoma, presence of a bleb after glaucoma filtering surgery, steroid-induced ocular hypertension, diabetic retinopathy requiring laser therapy, retinal vascular disease and sunken eyes or eyes with a narrow palpebral fissure. It is also important to record any previous ocular surgery (including refractive surgery) and ocular trauma. The patients should be asked to discontinue the use of any periocular cosmetics (especially eyeliners), 2 weeks prior to the surgery.

Systemic diseases such as diabetes, hypertension, heart disease, asthma, arthritis, etc. should be excluded. Specific enquiry into systemic vascular and autoimmune diseases is essential, as these are likely to affect wound healing. The medications (especially hormones and systemic steroids) that the patient is taking and any history of allergy should be noted.

Expectations

Inappropriate and unrealistic expectations from any refractive procedure are the most common causes of dissatisfaction after surgery. It is imperative that the patient understands that no refractive surgical procedure is perfect and an absolute correction may be impossible to achieve. The aim of the surgery is to decrease the dependence on spectacles or contact lenses, and it may not be possible to achieve a 20/20 unaided visual acuity. The need for a second surgical procedure should be explained to patients with high myopia and astigmatism, where regression may be a frequent problem. The patient should also understand the likely impact of surgery on the quality of his or her life, if a complication arises. For example, a temporary loss of best corrected acuity may prevent him or her legally driving a car for a period of time. In addition abnormalities in night vision and the immediate need for reading glasses in presbyopic patients needs to be emphasised. These are important issues that need to be discussed with the patients. Presbyopes should be counselled carefully and given the option for monovision.

<table>
<tr><td colspan="2" align="center">PATIENT EXCLUSION CRITERIA</td></tr>
<tr><td>1.</td><td>Ectatic corneal disease</td></tr>
<tr><td>2.</td><td>Thin corneas (< 450 μm)</td></tr>
<tr><td>3.</td><td>Active ocular infection</td></tr>
<tr><td>4.</td><td>Dry eye</td></tr>
<tr><td>5.</td><td>Glaucoma (especially if a large bleb is present)</td></tr>
<tr><td>6.</td><td>Blepharophimosis</td></tr>
<tr><td>7.</td><td>Monocular patients</td></tr>
<tr><td>8.</td><td>Large pupil size</td></tr>
<tr><td>9.</td><td>Systemic or retinal vascular disorder</td></tr>
<tr><td>10.</td><td>Autoimmune disease</td></tr>
<tr><td>11.</td><td>Pregnancy</td></tr>
</table>

CLINICAL EXAMINATION

The following are the salient features of the preoperative clinical evaluation of a patient who is to undergo LASIK.

Uncorrected and Best Corrected Visual Acuity (BCVA)

Uncorrected visual acuity (UCVA) both for near and distance should be recorded for all patients including those with high refractive errors. The appropriate correction is then put in the trial frame and the BCVA is measured. In moderate and high myopia, the BCVA may be measured using a soft or preferably hard contact lens, having a spherical equivalent as close as possible to that of the patient's refraction. Internally or externally illuminated visual acuity charts are best for this purpose. For accurate and meaningful statistical evaluation, the number of letters in each line of a LOGMAR chart read by the patient, should be recorded.

Manifest and Cycloplegic Refraction

The refraction is to be carefully performed with the aim of using the minimal myopic correction to provide the best visual acuity. The fellow eye is fogged with plus lenses and a duochrome test is performed to minimise the risk of overcorrection in myopes. For a more accurate estimation of the refraction at the corneal plane, the vertex distance must be measured in refractive errors of more than 4 diopters and a contact lens used to determine the manifest refraction and the BCVA. The new generation excimer laser machines make a correction for the vertex distance and thus do not require the optometrist to correct for the vertex distance. The actual refraction at the spectacle plane is directly fed into the computer of the excimer laser machine. In the event of any inconsistency, the refraction is to be repeated. To negate the effect of accommodation and over-estimation of myopia, a cycloplegic refraction is also required. One drop of 1 percent cyclopentolate or tropicamide given twice, 10 minutes apart, produces optimal cycloplegia, for a refraction within 30 to 40 minutes. Cylindrical errors should be expressed in minus form, so that the axis corresponds with the axis of the cylindrical ablation performed by the laser. It is the manifest refraction which forms the basis of the refractive surgery correction.

Fundus Examination

In all patients undergoing LASIK surgery, a cycloplegic refraction is performed. Concurrent mydriasis enables the refractive surgeon to undertake fundus examination with emphasis on peripheral retinal screening using the indirect ophthalmoscope. This is especially important in myopes because of the risk of an associated retinal pathology predisposing to a retinal detachment and the high stress on the vitreous base during application of firm pressure with the suction plate of the microkeratome. A suspicious lesion should be treated with laser or cryotherapy and the refractive surgery postponed for 6 to 8 weeks.

Slit-lamp Biomicroscopy

Before undertaking LASIK surgery, the anterior segment of the eye should be thoroughly examined to rule out various diseases that could result in adverse or suboptimal outcomes. The eyelids, conjunctiva, cornea, anterior chamber and lens should be systematically examined to exclude conditions such as blepharitis, dry eyes, corneal scars, keratoconus, corneal dystrophies or degenerations, iridocyclitis and cataract.

Keratometry

The power and axis of the steepest and flattest meridian of the cornea is determined by keratometry (Fig. 4.1). Keratometry is performed to determine the axis and magnitude of the corneal component of the astigmatism. It can also detect irregular astigmatism which characterises subclinical keratoconus. Keratometry readings should be used in conjunction with the corneal topography. The possibility of a free flap increases with a flat cornea (K < 40 D) and the possibility of a buttonhole is more in a steep cornea (K > 46 D). Such patients should be warned about the increased risk of microkeratome related complications.

Corneal Topography

Videokeratography (Figs 4.2 to 4.4) is an indispensable investigative tool to detect preoperative corneal diseases such as subclinical keratoconus, which is a contraindication for LASIK surgery. It also helps to determine irregularities on the corneal surface caused by contact lenses and to monitor the topographic

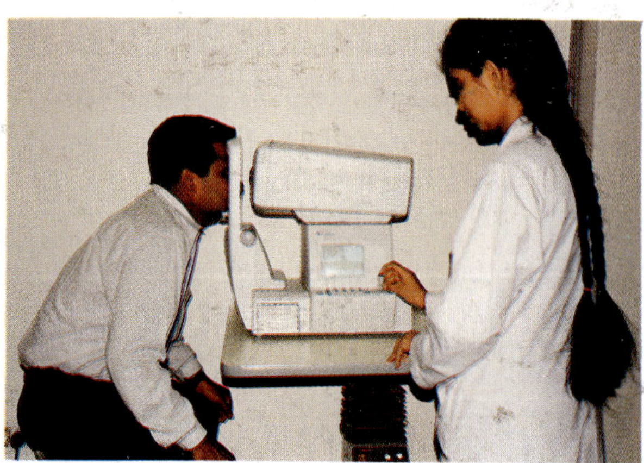

Fig. 4.1: Autokeratometry

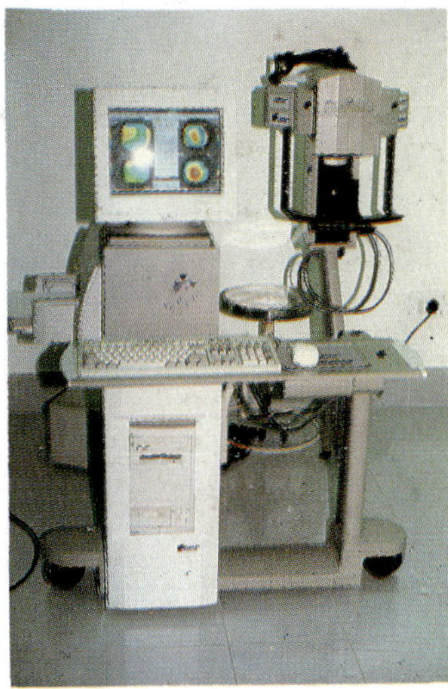

Fig. 4.2: Orbscan corneal topography system

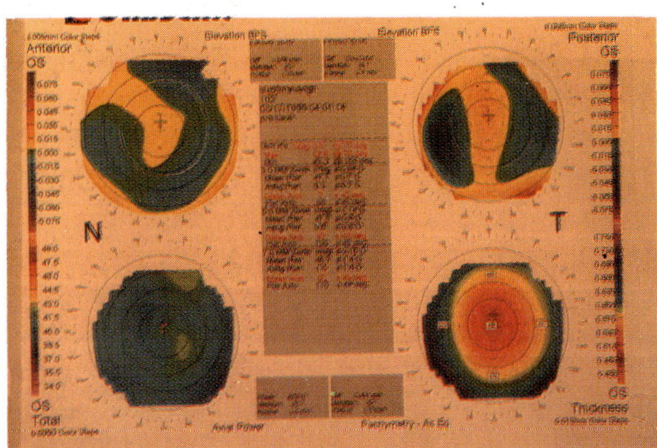

Fig. 4.3: Orbscan videokeratography showing the anterior best fit sphere (upper left), posterior best fit sphere (upper right), keratometric profile (lower left) and pachymetry (lower right)

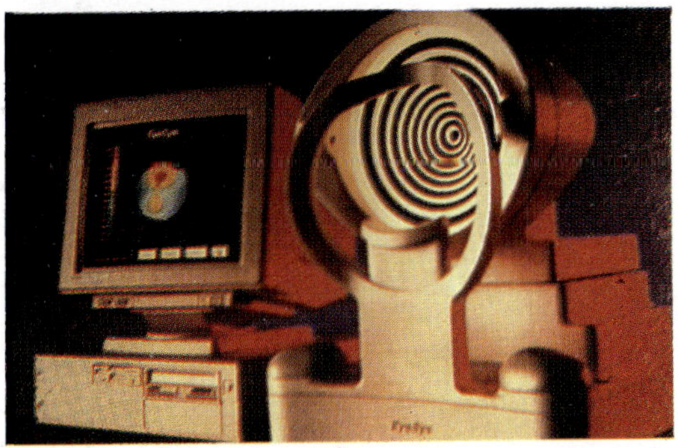

Fig. 4.4: Eyesys corneal topography system

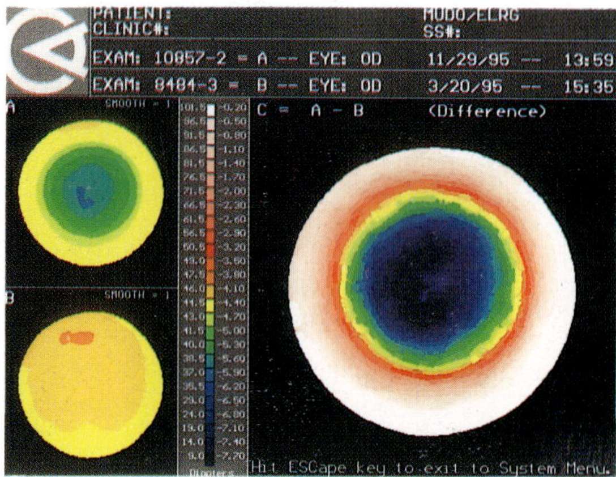

Fig. 4.5: Topography map after LASIK depicting central
blue zone of corneal flattening

changes after contact lens removal. The determination of the axis of corneal astigmatism is also aided by this investigation.

Corneal mapping by videokeratography is also an important tool to assess the efficacy of LASIK surgery (Fig. 4.5). It allows the refractive surgeon to comparatively evaluate preoperative and postoperative corneal maps in terms of corneal curvature and its dioptric power. The effect of the corneal ablation can be studied by comparing preoperative and postoperative maps taken at different times by using 'subtraction' or 'difference' maps. When this is done serially, one can start to visualise the changes in the tissue that has been ablated by looking at the 'difference' between the preoperative and the postoperative maps. The effect of wound healing (either epithelial, stromal, or both) can be seen comparing the initial postoperative difference map with the difference maps obtained at subsequent visits. In each case, the preoperative map is used as the standard or reference map. Decentration of the ablation, irregular astigmatism, central islands and corneal ectasia after LASIK are also picked up on corneal topography.

Topography-assisted LASIK (TA-LASIK) or topography-linked LASIK (TOPOLINK) is a new technique of refractive surgery in which the individual topography of a patient is used to custom- tailor the ablation, such that the cornea can be reshaped in any manner we choose. The topography of the patient is electronically transferred on to the computer of the excimer laser machine. This system uses a new software which converts the measurements of the radii of curvature obtained on the topography map into true height values, based on which the ablation is calculated. The target keratometry and the diameter of the desired ablation zone have to be fed in by the surgeon. The computer then calculates a specific treatment profile based on the corneal topography of the individual patient. The TOPOLINK system is especially useful in the treatment of irregular astigmatism

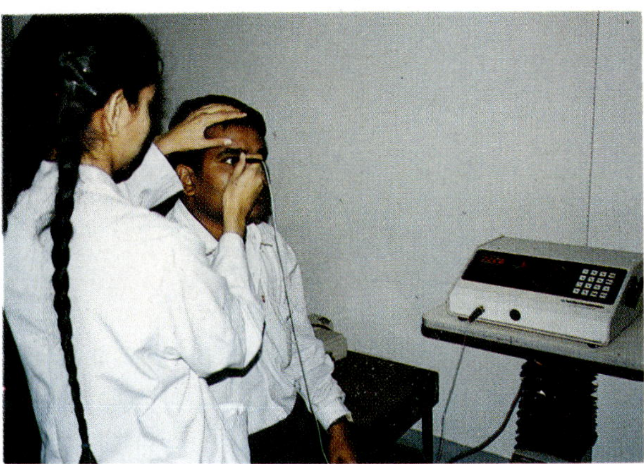

Fig. 4.6: Ultrasonic pachymetry

and residual refractive errors following penetrating keratoplasty, radial keratotomy, cataract surgery and corneal injuries.

Pachymetry

Estimation of corneal thickness by using an ultrasonic pachymeter is essential prior to LASIK surgery (Fig. 4.6). It helps in determining the thickness of central cornea, the thickness of the flap and the amount of corneal tissue available for a safe and effective corneal stromal ablation. This is particularly important in treatments for high and extreme myopes and in retreatments where a treatment algorithm has to be designed in such a way that an adequate residual stromal thickness 250 µm (although some surgeons may use 200 µm as the minimum residual thickness) is ensured after the ablation. Pachymetry is performed centrally, but may also be done at 3, 5, and 7 mm paracentrally. It has been seen that the optical pachymetry incorporated into corneal topography systems (such as the Orbscan) gives a much higher value as compared to ultrasonic pachymetry.

Some surgeons also do an intraoperative pachymetry to assess the thickness of the flap created by the microkeratome and the residual thickness of the stromal bed, before and after the ablation. Special pachymeters have been developed to measure the corneal epithelial thickness after LASIK. This helps to ascertain epithelial hyperplasia after the surgery which is an important cause for regression after LASIK.

Pupil Size

This is an important part of the examination and is often neglected. Since glare and haloes can cause a significant handicap in dim illumination, especially during night driving, the pupil size should be measured under both mesopic and scotopic light conditions. The infrared pupillometer is an ideal device for such

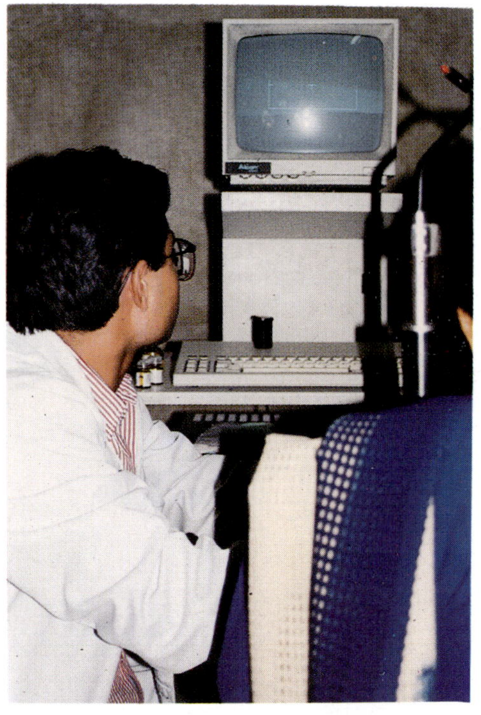

Fig. 4.7: Specular microscopy of the corneal endothelium

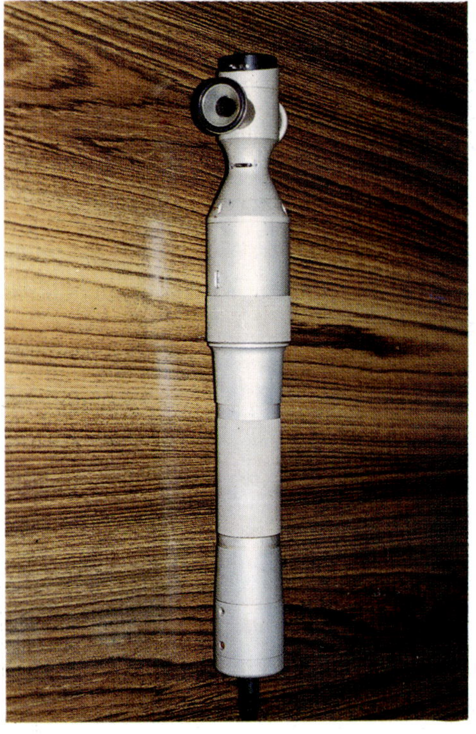

Fig. 4.8: Hand-held glare tester

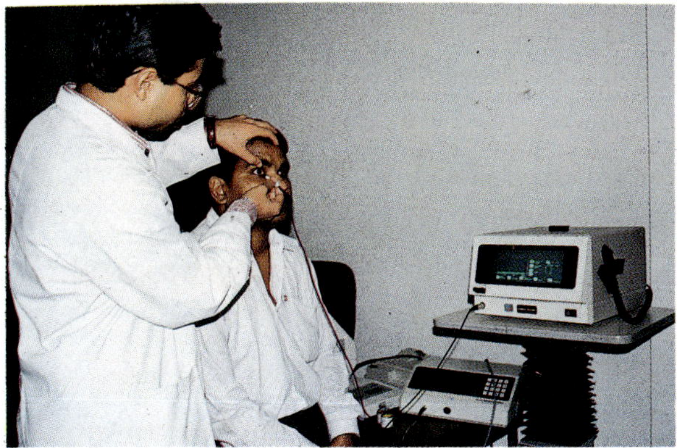

Fig. 4.9: Ultrasonic biometry

measurements. If this instrument is not available, then a simple pupil gauge can be used.

The evaluation of eye exposure, intraocular pressure (IOP), corneal endothelial specular microscopy (Fig. 4.7), glare (Fig. 4.8), contrast sensitivity and ocular biometry (Fig. 4.9) are some of the other tests to be conducted before the refractive procedure.

PREOPERATIVE EXAMINATION

1. Uncorrected and best corrected visual acuity
2. Cycloplegic, subjective and manifest refraction
3. Slit-lamp biomicroscopy
4. Fundus examination
5. Keratometry
6. Corneal topography
7. Pachymetry
8. Pupil size
9. Glare and contrast sensitivity
10. Specular microscopy
11. Biometry (axial length)
12. Tonometry

Five

Microkeratomes for LASIK

The microkeratome is the basic instrument required to make a corneal flap, to facilitate intrastromal excimer laser ablation during LASIK. The purpose of the microkeratome is to create a uniform and homogeneous corneal flap of a precisely calculated diameter and thickness, by cutting across the stromal corneal lamellae. The cutting action of the microkeratome is derived from a blade which is powered by an electromechanical system (or turbine system). The microkeratome motor is powered through a cable and activated by a foot pedal control. The following components are included in an assembled microkeratome

Head — contains the thickness plate, blade holder and blade
Handle — contains the motor
Footplate — to stabilize and pressurise the eye
Console — for power control.

An ideal microkeratome should be simple to assemble and operate, easy to clean and reassemble or readily disposable, allow visibility of the cornea during creation of the flap and demonstrate dependability, durability and repeatability in several consecutive cases.

A number of different microkeratomes have been developed by various scientists around the world and are available for clinical use (Table 5.1). There are several more microkeratomes referred to in the literature, that are still under development and not in commercial use. The following section gives a brief description of the various microkeratomes used for LASIK.

BARRAQUER MICROKERATOME

Jose Ignacio Barraquer designed the original microkeratome that served as the basis for the development of all subsequent microkeratomes. Barraquer's original microkeratome consisted of a head with a steel blade that was passed manually over the cornea. The system had the following components:

Blade

It is a precision surgical blade with a dot marked on its surface to indicate the correct orientation, since it can be mounted only in one way onto the blade holder.

The rear of the blade contains a groove that must face posteriorly to engage the eccentric pin of the motor, providing oscillatory movement with a lateral excursion of approximately 2.5 mm of the blade holder and blade.

Plate

The thickness plate is made of plastic or stainless steel. It allows the surgeon to set the depth of the lamellar cut. These plates are available in multiple thickness and can be changed to give flaps of the required thickness. The thickness plate is fitted in a specific groove situated in the anterior portion of the microkeratome head. With traditional microkeratomes, the absence of the plate or its incorrect insertion into the head of the microkeratome could cause a full-thickness cut through the cornea. Such a perforating injury could lead to damage of the iris and the lens and even vitreous loss. Although every step in the assembly of the microkeratome is important, the proper fitting of the thickness plate is of vital importance.

Suction Ring

A suction ring is an integral part of the microkeratome. Besides helping in fixing the eyeball and raising the intraocular pressure (IOP) to facilitate creation of the corneal flap, it contains a track which engages the microkeratome and allows the surgeon to regulate the accurate movement of the microkeratome. The suction plate is made up of steel and the original microkeratome had 10 different sized rings for different diameter corneal cuts. The newer microkeratomes utilise a single suction ring and different diameters of corneal tissue are cut by adjusting the height of the ring. The suction ring has a hollow handle to which a silicone tube is attached to transmit suction from the suction pump in the console. To achieve an ideal cut, the suction should increase the IOP to 60 to 65 mm Hg. This needs to be carefully checked with an applanation tonometer before using the microkeratome. Inadequate suction will result in an irregular, thin flap or a buttonhole.

AUTOMATED CORNEAL SHAPER

Automated Corneal Shaper (ACS) has been designed by Luis Ruiz and is produced by Chiron Vision Inc (Fig. 5.1). Although it is fundamentally similar to the Barraquer's microkeratome, the key difference is that it has an automated advancement mechanism that acts through a gear system to advance the blade in a uniform and regular way. It is available in two forms: combined ALK/LASIK unit which can cut flaps of varying thickness and diameter and the dedicated LASIK unit which is preset. The ACS has the following parts:

Shaper head

The microkeratome head houses the blade which is driven by an electric motor at a rate of 8000 rpm. The side of the shaper head has three gears that constitute

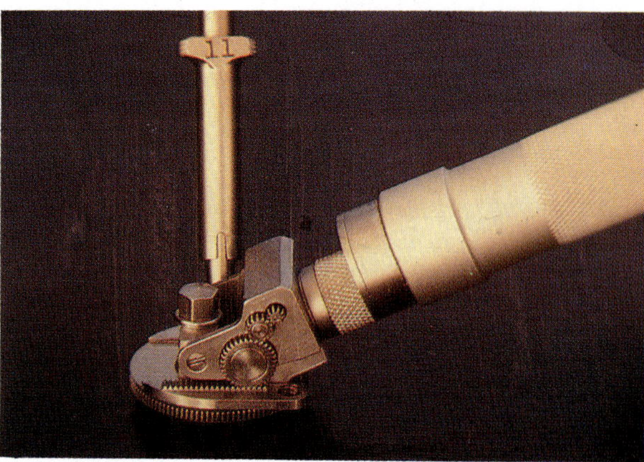

Fig. 5.1: Chiron automated corneal shaper

the core of the instrument's automated movement system. These gears are driven by the electric motor in the handle that also operates the oscillating blade. The first gear transmits a rotatory impulse to the other two gears and engages a gear track on the suction ring, thereby, driving the microkeratome across the cornea. A stopper mechanism has been incorporated in the shaper head to limit the complete run of the microkeratome along the track. This leaves an incomplete hinged flap rather than a free flap. The depth of the corneal cut is controlled by the thickness plate that is fitted in the designated groove, on the anterior portion of shaper head. These plates are numbered progressively and the thickness of the plate used determines the thickness of the corneal flap. If a thin plate is used, the space between plate and the blade would be larger allowing a greater exposure of the corneal tissue to the microkeratome, and this will create a thicker flap. For LASIK, a plate which allows creation of a 160 μm thick corneal flap is employed.

Motor

The motor of the microkeratome is a 12-volt micromotor that is housed in a cylindrical handle. This handle connects to the posterior aspect of the shaper head and drives both the oscillating blade and the gears. The motor is connected through a cable to the control box. The motor is activated by a two-mode foot pedal that can be pressed for changing the direction of the direct current, for forward and backward movements of the microkeratome.

Pneumatic Fixation Ring

The suction ring serves primarily to stabilise the globe. Other uses of the ring include guiding the microkeratome to move on its gear track and facilitating smooth passage of the cutting blade, increasing the IOP prior to the cutting of the cornea and determining the position of the flap. The ring is made up of steel and has a rectangular chamber on its underside. This chamber is connected to a suction pump in the control unit, through the tubing attached to the handle of the suction ring. The suction pump creates a vacuum within the chamber. The optimal vacuum for LASIK is in the range of 22 to 27 mm Hg.

Control Unit

The control unit contains the suction pump for the pneumatic suction ring and provides the power to both the suction pump and motor of the microkeratome. On the front panel of the control unit, there are two metres to show the levels of vacuum created in the suction ring and amplitude of power delivered to the motor of the microkeratome. The voltage metre indicates the power delivered for the advancement and reversal of the microkeratome (optimal requirement is 12 volts).

Foot Pedal

Two separate foot pedals are supplied with the control unit – a suction pedal and a power pedal. To initiate and maintain the suction, the suction pump is activated by simply depressing and releasing the suction pedal. After the completion of the LASIK procedure, the suction is disengaged and the pneumatic ring released by pressing and releasing the suction pedal for a second time. The power pedal has two parts – one to activate and advance the microkeratome across the cornea to create the corneal flap, and the other to reverse the microkera-tome after the completion of the corneal cut.

SCHWIND MICROKERATOME

The Schwind microkeratome is produced by Herbert Schwind and has been designed and developed by Hoffmann and Seiler (Fig. 5.2). This microkeratome

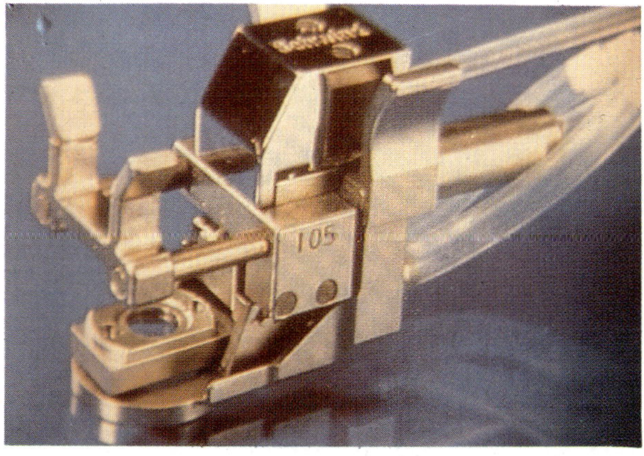

Fig. 5.2: Schwind microkeratome

is different from traditional microkeratomes such as the ACS and has the following design characteristics:

- The device comes as a single unit with accompanying power pack and foot controls.
- The microkeratome blade is reusable and is made up of sapphire. Each blade can be used approximately for 400 cuts. The angle of contact of the blade with the cornea is 0 degree as compared to 26 degree angle of other microkeratomes, which allows for a low oscillation speed (1600 – 1800 rpm) during the cut.
- The blade is electrically propelled and its progression is automated. Its movement is straight and harmonic. The progression speed of the blade is 1.33 mm/sec for a total of 6 seconds. The thickness plate is fixed and only allows corneal cuts of 150 μm depth. Both anterior and posterior parts of the plate are transparent and the surgeon can directly view the action of the blade on the corneal tissue during the entire procedure.
- The vacuum system of the unit contains two suction rings. The rings are fixed and non-adjustable. One ring fixes the eyeball in the peripheral cornea and the other stabilises the corneal flap during the incision
- The electrical motor system of the device is situated in the instrument's console and two metal drive cables transmit the advancing and oscillatory movements of the blade.
- This microkeratome cuts a 150 μm thick flap of 9 mm diameter with 0.5 mm hinge.

The disadvantages of this keratome are the marked vibrations of the instrument, the low oscillation speed of the blade and the use of metal cables to transmit power.

TURBOKERATOME (SCMD MICROKERATOME)

Under the aegis of SCMD Ltd. this turbine microkeratome has been developed by John Livecchi. It has the following characteristics (Fig. 5.3):

- The microkeratome head is fixed and does not have a thickness plate. The microkeratome produces a fixed 150 μm flap thickness
- There is a bifaceted blade made up of metal. The angle of attack on the cornea is 20 degrees and its oscillating cycles range from 10,000 to 24,000 rpm, although the recommended oscillation speed of operation is 13,800 rpm. The direction of blade movement is sideways.
- The microkeratome is independent of electrical power and the oscillations of the blade are powered by a turbine with nitrogen protoxide propulsion.
- The microkeratome does not have an automated progression system and is advanced manually by the surgeon.
- A digital micrometer with adjustment screws between the handle and the head of the microkeratome permits the surgeon to set the stop point and therefore determine the length of the cut.

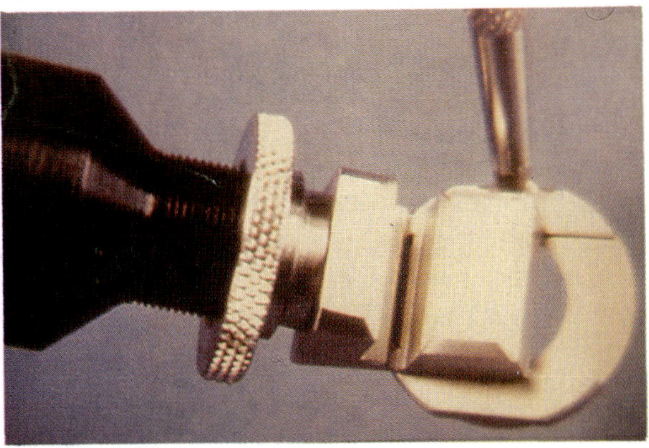

Fig. 5.3: Turbokeratome with suction ring

- The unit has multiple suction rings and can create flaps of varying diameter and there are four stop rings that give varying hinge dimensions.

UNIVERSAL KERATOME

The Universal keratome (Fig. 5.4) has been developed by Phoenix Keratek Inc. of Scottsdale under the guidance of Perry S Binder. The keratome has the following innovative features
- The microkeratome comes as a single unit and has a suction ring incorporated in it. There are no separate handled suction rings.
- The thickness plate and suction ring are fixed and provide only a hinged flap of preset thickness and diameter.
- The metal blade is unifaceted and its attack angle on to the cornea is 0 degree.

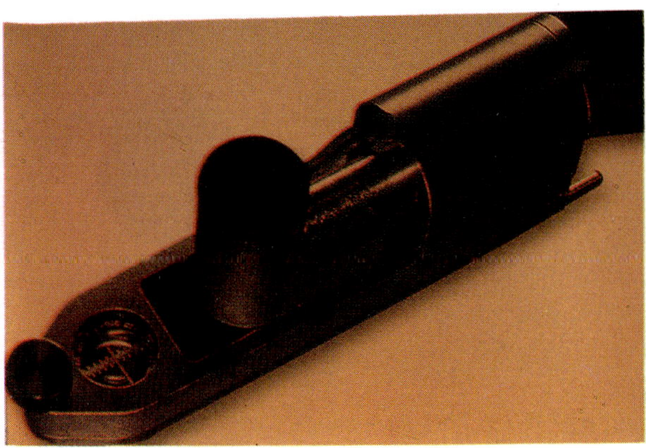

Fig. 5.4: Universal keratome

- The blade is powered by a piezoelectric motor and the blade oscillates at a speed of 14,000 rpm with a straight pendular movement.
- The device is automatically advanced using an electrical motor drive.
- The device has a computer controlled console to regulate the resistance and the cutting speed on the cornea.
- The system is unique in that it has a series of polymethylmethacrylate (PMMA) discs that can be used for refractive resections for the correction of myopia and hyperopia.
- The surgeon has a direct view of the corneal cutting during the procedure and can observe whether the cut has been performed correctly.

MASTEL-BUZARD MICROKERATOME

Mastel-Buzard microkeratome has been designed and developed by Mastel Precision Surgical Instruments Inc. under the guidance of David Mastel and Kurt Buzard. The microkeratome has the following specific features:
- The device is built as a single piece with integrated vacuum as a part of it.
- The unit has a diamond blade that is advanced manually by the surgeon.
- The microkeratome creates a hinged flap of a fixed diameter of 8.5 mm with the hinge being parallel to the eyebrow.
- The incision is created by advancing the diamond blade with the surgeon's thumb after engaging the cornea and then pushing the thumb piece to the stop, which completes the cut.

AUTOMATED DISPOSABLE KERATOME

Automated Disposable Keratome (Fig. 5.5) has been designed by Luis Antonio Ruiz and has been developed by Laser Sight Technologies Inc. The Automated Disposable Keratome has the following features:
- It comes as a preassembled, sterile packaged, single-use, moulded plastic device.
- The microkeratome has a vacuum safety ridge that can establish dual vacuum chambers to decrease the likelihood of vacuum port occlusion and false suction.
- The metal blade has a speed of 10,000 rpm and is advanced automatically.
- The thickness plates are an integral part of the head and cannot be removed. Two types of the devices are available for creation of flaps of either 130 µm or 160 µm.
- The gears of the device are covered to minimise the chances of entrapment of lids or lashes, or injury.
- The unit has a tandem track drive that can eliminate the torque seen in single track units.
- The components of the device are fabricated from transparent plastic, allowing the surgeon a direct view of the operative surface.
- The device can create both horizontal and vertical flaps.

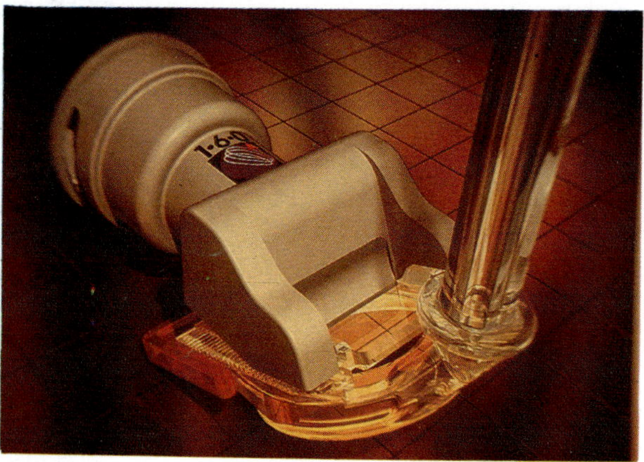

Fig. 5.5: Lasersight automated disposable keratome

The inherent disadvantage of all plastic microkeratomes is the generation of plastic debris, which settles on the cut surface of the stromal bed.

INNOVATOME

This microkeratome has been developed by Innovative Optics Inc (Fig. 5.6). Its distinctive design features are as follows:
- It is a lightweight, moulded plastic microkeratome, weighing only 37 gm on the eye.
- The microkeratome has an automated advancement system and is driven by a single flexible cable. There are no gears or mechanical assemblies.
- The unit has a disposable steel blade that is electrically driven and has a oscillation speed of 12,000 rpm.

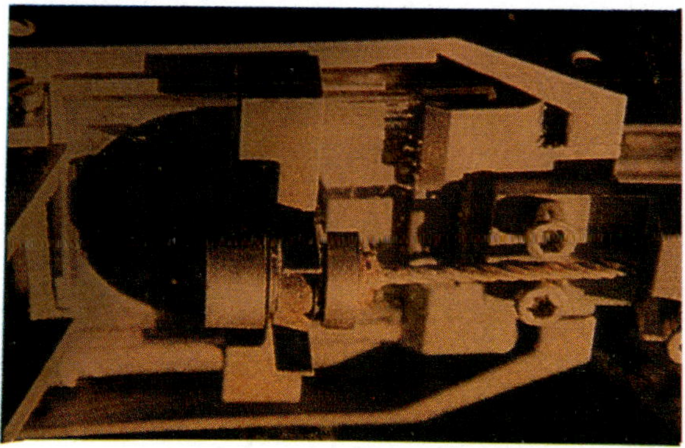

Fig. 5.6: Innovative optics innovatome

- The microkeratome allows the creation of either horizontal or vertical flaps. The flap diameter can range from 8.5 mm to 10 mm.
- The device has a clear sapphire applanator that allows the surgeon to directly view the operative field. The applanator is marked to enable the surgeon to predict the location of hinge.
- The pneumatic fixation ring is integrated in the device and is mechanically grooved to provide infinite points of suction.

MICROPRECISION'S MICROLAMELLAR KERATOME

This microkeratome system is distributed by Eye Technology Inc. The device has the following design characteristics:
- The unit has a metal blade that is bifaceted and angulated at 9 degrees. The blade drive has a sideways movement with 20,000 oscillations per minute.
- The blade drive is powered by a pneumatic turbine and has six times the torque of electric motors.
- The microkeratome is manually advanced by the surgeon.
- The device has an adjustable thickness plate which allows creation of a range of corneal flaps from 0 to 466 μm in 1 μm increments. The calibration of thickness plate is verified with a micrometer.
- The unit comes with multiple suction rings that allow for flaps of varying diameters.
- The suction rings and microkeratome head have dual dove-tail rail systems to create the flap which decreases the risk of jumping and causes fewer chatter marks in the stroma, leading to a smoother keratectomy bed.
- The device has a 'stop-pin' system to create a hinged flap but does not allow the surgeon to directly visualise the operative field.

SOLAN FLAPMAKER DISPOSABLE MICROKERATOME

This microkeratome is being manufactured and distributed by Refractive Technologies Inc, Cleveland, Ohio. The device has the following design features (Fig. 5.7):
- The device comes as a preassembled, single-use, moulded plastic unit and is completely disposable.
- The unit does not have any gears and is driven by flexible shafts that provide a uniform motion of the microkeratome.
- The device has a metal blade made from surgical stainless steel which has an oscillation speed of 12,500 cycles per minute. It is driven across the cornea at 6.8 mm per second and only oscillates in the forward motion.
- The resection depth is variable from 160 to 220 μm and the flap produced has a diameter of 10.5 mm.
- The unit is made of injection-moulded polycarbonate and allows the surgeon to directly visualise the operative field.

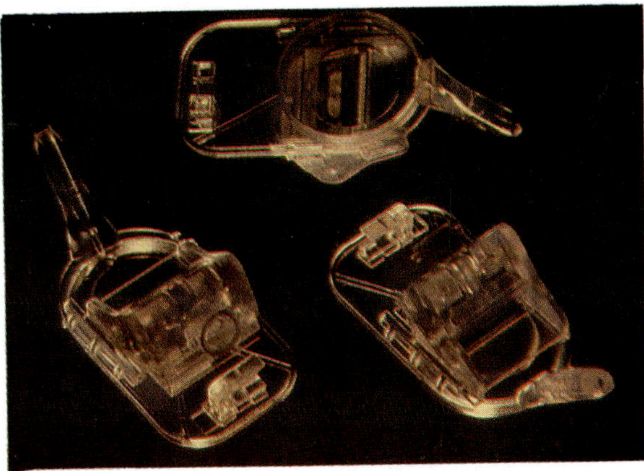

Fig. 5.7: Flapmaker disposable microkeratome

CLEAR CORNEAL MOLDER

Dr Ricardo Guimaraes of Brazil has developed this microkeratome for use in LASIK. The microkeratome has the following distinctive features:
- The device comes as a single-piece integrated instrument unit that includes the head with a dual axis motor, the handle, the suction ring and the plate.
- The device has a diamond or steel blade which is powered by an electrical motor and has an oscillation rate of 12,000 per minute with a 0 degree angle of attack on the cornea.
- The diameter and the thickness of the corneal flap cut by the device can be varied.
- The device has only one pneumatic fixation ring and the height is adjustable in relation to the blade.
- The device has a transparent surface and allows the surgeon to directly visualise the operative field during the surgery.

The blade movement can be stopped at a preset point with a lever on the handle of the microkeratome which allows both free caps or hinged flaps to be obtained.

LAMELLAR KERATOPLASTY SYSTEM (PLANCON INSTRUMENTS MICROKERATOME)

This device is manufactured by Plancon Instruments of Anatony, France and is distributed by Moria of France. It has the following features:
- It is a non-automated microkeratome in which the head is advanced manually.
- The device has a bifaceted metal blade that oscillates at 15,000 cycles per minute. The blade oscillations are powered by a turbine which is driven by nitrogen gas and the blade attack angle is 22.5 degrees.

- The microkeratome has four thickness plates allowing cut thickness of 120, 140, 160 and 180 μm.
- The unit comes with multiple suction rings depending on the diameter of the flap desired and the suction rings are less bulky as compared to other rings available, which is helpful to create an adequate exposure in eyes with a narrow palpebral fissure.
- There are four metal stop rings which enables the surgeon to create a corneal hinge of diameters ranging between 1.5 and 2.5 mm.
- An adjustable micrometer is located at the junction of the head and the handle, which limits the excursion of the keratome to the exact point as set by the surgeon.

MORIA LSK CARRIAZO-BARRAQUER MICROKERATOME

This is a popular keratome currently in use by many LASIK surgeons. The hand piece and the blades used are both made up of stainless steel. The functioning of this microkeratome may be manual or automated.

- The steel blade makes 14,000 oscillations per minute and advances at the rate of 3.7 mm/second. The blade angle is 30 degree.
- The microkeratome can cut a flap of diameter ranging between 7 mm and 10.5 mm.
- Multiple suction rings are provided and the depth of the cut is precalibrated at 160 μm or 180 μm.
- A variable flap orientation is possible with this microkeratome.
- An electric motor is the power source in the automated machine, while the manual keratome functions on the nitrogen gas turbine.

MORIA LSK ONE DISPOSABLE

This a manual disposable microkeratome manufactured by Moria Inc. and uses a plastic hand piece technology (Fig. 5.8).

- A stainless steel blade with a blade angle of 25 degree and an oscillation rate of 14,000 per minute is incorporated in the instrument.
- The flap created by this microkeratome can vary in diameter between 7 mm and 10 mm.
- Multiple suction rings are provided for eye fixation and the depth of the cut is preset at 160 μm or 180 μm.
- A variable flap orientation is possible with this keratome and the power source is derived from a nitrogen gas turbine.

ML MICROKERATOME (A and M)

The Med-Logics microkeratome may be automated (A) or manual (M). It is made up of a titanium hand piece and uses stainless steel blades to create the flap. It runs on an electric power source.

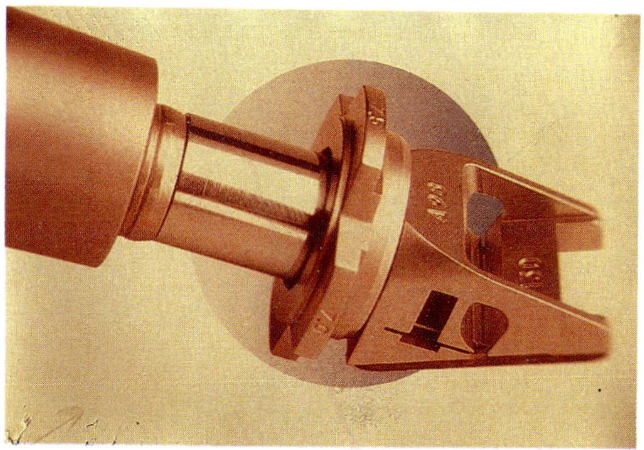

Fig. 5.8: Moria LSK-one microkeratome

- The blade angle is 24 degrees, the oscillation frequency varies between 9000 and 15,000 oscillations per minute and the rate of advancement of the blade is 3.5 to 5.0 mm/sec.
- The diameter of the flap created by this microkeratome is between 8 mm and 10 mm and the flap orientation is variable.
- Two suction rings are provided and the depth of the flap created is 160 μm or 180 μm.

MICRATOME ADVANCED REFRACTIVE INSTRUMENTATION

The MICRA **ACRI** microkeratome is a manual instrument and the currently available model is Model 7000. The hand piece is made up of titanium or steel (Fig. 5.9).

- A stainless steel blade cartridge is used as the cutting mechanism and the blade angle is 25 degrees.
- Nitrogen gas is used as the power source and the oscillation speed of the blade is 15,000 oscillations per minute.
- A universal suction ring is provided and the depth of the flap can be 130, 160 or 200 μm.
- The flap diameter is variable up to 10 mm but the flap orientation is fixed.

HANSATOME

The Hansatome (Fig. 5.10) has been developed by Chiron Vision Corp. It is a device that further refines the ability of the ACS devised by Ruiz and is currently a popular microkeratome for LASIK. The microkeratome has the following design characteristics:

- The microkeratome head has a fixed depth plate and a permanent non-adjustable stop device.

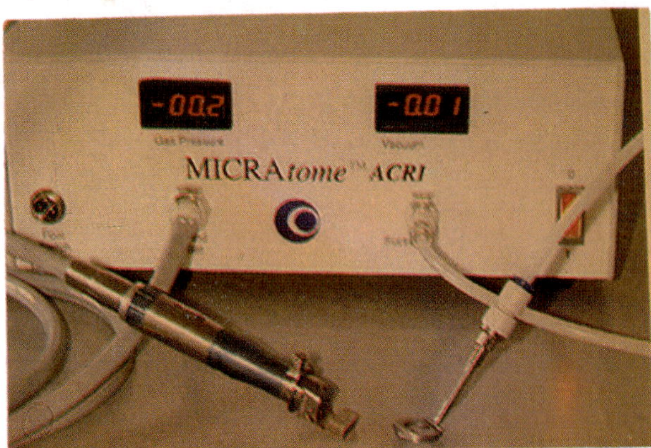

Fig. 5.9: ACRI microkeratome (MICRA)

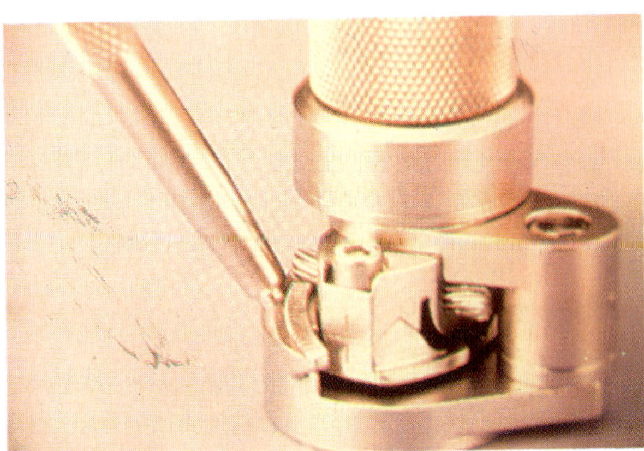

Fig. 5.10: Chiron Hansatome microkeratome

- The device utilises a disposable metal blade and comes with an integrated plastic holder.
- The unit has two suction rings (8.5 mm and 9.5 mm) that have an elevated, curved gear rack that aligns with the single gear of the Hansatome.
- The Hansatome creates a superiorly placed hinge at 12 o'clock position which can be protected by the upper lid.
- Two heads with fixed thickness plates are provided which cut flaps of preset thickness:160 μm and 180 μm.
- There is a left/right eye adapter that fits over the microkeratome head and the motor is positioned vertically,which enables the microkeratome head to pass over the suction ring on an elevated track away from the speculum and the eyelids.

- The cutting action of the microkeratome cannot be started until the appropriate vacuum level is reached and the cutting stops if the vacuum falls below a certain level.

The important points to remember before placing it on the eye are
- Inspection of the blade under the microscope
- Inspection of the head and gears for debris
- Check the fitting of the motor head
- Visually confirm the blade oscillation
- Inspection of the suction ring and cleaning of debris
- Inspection of the suction ports to verify that they are open
- Verify full microkeratome pass before placing it on the eye
- Use a new blade for each eye.

VISIJET HYDROKERATOME

This keratome uses a *Water jet* technology to create a *cleavage* in between the corneal lamellae. This is accomplished by fatiguing and breaking the collagen bonds between the corneal lamellae while preserving the integrity of the lamellae and the keratocytes. Since the cornea is a highly sectile tissue, cleavage rather than cutting is the best mechanism for tissue separation with minimal tissue damage. Therefore this procedure is less traumatic and much safer as compared to the mechanical microkeratomes which cut across the corneal tissues. The anticipated advantages of the hydrokeratome are a decrease in epithelial ingrowth, irregular astigmatism, haze, regression and flap or suction related complications.

The Visijet hydrokeratome (Fig. 5.11) uses a continuous beam of ultrahigh pressure saline that is only 36 microns in diameter, to cut a flap across the cornea.

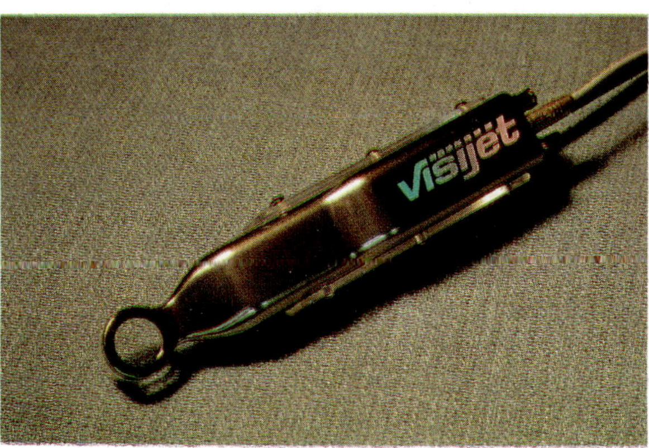

Fig. 5.11: Visijet hydrokeratome

The key to the hydrokeratome's success is the extreme high pressure (over 15,000 psi) combined with a tightly collimated water jet beam. Under these "ultrafluidic conditions" the water molecules leave the orifice of the instrument at a speed in excess of 800 mph and take on almost metallic properties. The device has the following design features:

- The device uses a high pressure water-jet beam to cleave the cornea.
- The surgeon controlled foot switch activates the suction ring vacuum, the water jet aspiration and the high pressure water jet beam.
- A hand piece translates the water jet across the cornea. The angle of attack of the water beam on the cornea is 0 degree.
- The end point of water jet operation is preprogrammed by the surgeon depending on the selected hinge length and flap diameter.
- The water pressure and water jet beam position are continuously monitored by an image tracking technology.
- The flap thickness can be varied from 100 to 200 microns, depending on the thickness plate used. The flap diameter ranges from 8 to 11 mm.
- The applanating surface is made up of lexan, a special plastic and has a diameter of 12 mm. The surface is transparent and the surgeon has a full visualisation of the visual axis at all times.

Since this keratome is easy to use, has a low cost and an increased safety, this is expected to gain wide acceptance among LASIK surgeons in the coming years.

MEDJET HYDROBLADE KERATOME

This is also an automated keratome based on the water jet technology. It uses a circular water beam to create a lamellar corneal flap. The flap diameter is adjustable up to 9 mm. The eye fixation is done by a single suction ring at a normal IOP. The depth of the cut is adjustable but the orientation of the flap cannot be varied. The power source for this hydrokeratome is a pneumatic pump.

LASER MICROKERATOME

This is the microkeratome of the future, still under development. The **IntraLase Femtosecond Laser Microkeratome** and the **Novatec Laser Microkeratome** are are examples of two such laser keratomes. The laser microkeratome is used as an intrastromal cutting tool based on picosecond intrastromal photodisruption. It causes separation and removal of a small amount of stromal collagen from within the cornea by focusing highly transmissive infrared laser light through the cornea. The main advantages of this technique are the precision and reproducibility of the laser in producing flaps of uniform thickness and the smoothness of the flap interface. Suction rings and the cutting blades are also not required in this procedure. Currently, the limitations of this laser technology are the small flap diameter, poor centration, increased intraoperative time and difficulty in dissection. Research is on to develop a solid state ultraviolet laser which can be used both for cutting the flap and intrastromal ablation.

Table 5.1: Microkeratomes for LASIK

Microkeratome	Function	Cutting mechanism	Blade angle	Oscillations per minute	Advance rate	Flap diameter	Flap Depth
Conventional Bausch and Lomb surgical Automated corneal shaper	Automatic	Stainless steel blade	26°	8,000	3.7 mm/sec	Variable up to 9.0 mm	160 μm
Bausch and Lomb surgical Hansatome Microkeratome	Automatic	Stainless steel blade	25°	NS	NS	Fixed at 8.5 or 9.5 mm	160 μm or 180 μm
Herbert Schwind Supratome	Both	Stainless steel blade	30°	11,000	16.6°/sec	7.0-10.0 mm	160 μm or 180 μm
Innovative Optics Innovatome	Automatic	Stainless steel blade	NS	24,000	1.0-4.0 mm/sec	8.9-9.2 mm (myopia) 9.4-9.6 mm (hyperopia)	130, 160 or 190 μm
Mastel Precision Surgical Instuments Buzard diamond Barraqueratome	Manual or automatic	Crystal diamond	> 50°	0	Adjustable	9.1 mm (myopia) 10.0 mm (hyperopic)	Fixed at 160 μm
Med-logics ML Microkeratome A	Automatic	Stainless steel blade	24°	9,000-15,000	3.5-5.0 mm/sec	8.0-10.0 mm	160 μm, 180 μm
Micra Micratome Advanced Corneal/Refractive Instrumentation (ACRI) Modal 7000	Manual	Stainless steel blade cartridge	25°	Variable	NA up to 15,000	Up to 10.0 mm	130 μm, 160 μm, 200 μm
Moria LSK one	Manual	Stainless steel blade	25°	14,000	NA	7.0-10.0 mm	Precalibrated: 130 μm, 160 μm, 180 μm
Moria LSK Carriazo-Barraquer	Manual or Automatic	Stainless steel blade	30°	14,000	3.7 mm/sec (automatic)	7.0-10.5 mm	Precalibrated: 160, 180 μm
New United Development Corp Turbokeratome (SCMD)	Manual	Stainless steel blade	25°	15,000	NA	Variable up to 10.0 mm	130-150 μm
Summit Krumeich-Barraquer Microkeratome	Automatic	Steel blade	26°	1-20,000 rpm	0.1-3.0 mm/sec	8.0-10.0 mm	130, 160, 180 μm

Contd...

Table contd..

Microkeratome	Function	Cutting mechanism	Blade angle	Oscillations per minute	Advance rate	Flap diameter	Flap Depth
Disposable Katena Products Inc Barron Microkeratome	Manual	Stainless steel blade	25°	20,000	NA	8.5 or 9.5 mm	160 µm
Laser sight-Automated disposable Keratome	Automatic	Stainless steel blade	26°	10,000	4.5 mm/sec	8.5-9.5 mm	130 or 160 µm
Moria LSK one disposable	Manual	Stainless steel blade	25°	14,000	NA	7.0-10.0 mm	Precalibrated: 160, 180 µm
Solan ophthalmic products Flapmaker	Automatic	Stainless steel blade	26°	12,500	6.8 mm/sec	8.5 mm or 10.5 mm	130-220 µm
Water jet Medjet hydroblade keratome	Automatic	Circular water beam	NA	NA	NA	Adjustable up to 9.0 mm	Adjustable
Visijet hydrokeratome	Automatic	Water beam	NA	NA	6.7 mm/sec	7.0-11.0 mm	120-200 µm
Laser Intralase femtoecond laser Microkeratome	Automatic	Laser photodisruption	NA	NA	NA	10.0 mm	Variable
Novatec laser microkeratome	Automatic	Transmissive wavelength Laser	NA	NA	NA	Creates intrastromal bubbles and flaps	Infinitely adjustable

NA – Not applicatble
NS – Not supplied by company

Care and Maintenance of the Microkeratome

The microkeratome must be cleaned immediately and thoroughly after each use. Failure to do so can result in residual debris, drying and sticking onto the microkeratome components. If the components are then autoclaved, this debris may become firmly attached onto the components. Debris along the track of the microkeratome can interfere in the smooth movement of the keratome and lead to serious flap-related complications. To remove the debris, the components should be soaked in hot distilled water for a minimum of 15 minutes, and then cleaned with a special solution as mentioned in the manufacturer's manual. A medium bristle toothbrush should be employed to scrub all the instruments while using the special cleaning solution. All components must be thoroughly rinsed with distilled water after cleaning in the solution and immediately dried with a lint-free surgical wipe or with microfiltered air. To minimise the creation of debris, distilled water should be used during the surgery to irrigate the stromal bed. The use of any type of salt solution can lead to accumulation of the salt crystals in the microkeratome and the gear track.

The motor of the instrument, the motor cord, the power/suction unit and the vacuum & motor foot switch should not be immersed in any fluid. A cloth moistened with isopropyl alcohol should be used to wipe the surfaces of each of these devices. The shaft of the motor should be cleaned with a dry toothbrush.

Six

Laser Delivery Systems

It is important to understand the basic features of the excimer laser delivery systems, which are commercially available for application in refractive surgery. The rapid technological advancements have lead to the improvement in these delivery systems with incorporation of an updated software, sophisticated scanning and eye tracking systems. Each system has a specific ablation approach with inherent advantages and disadvantages. The three major delivery systems being used are:

1. Wide field ablation
2. Scanning slit ablation
3. Flying spot ablation.

Wide Field Ablation

The principle feature of the wide field ablation delivery system is the use of a stationary, broad and circular beam of the excimer laser for corneal tissue removal. This is the first generation laser delivery system and has got the longest track record. Since a broad beam is used, the exact alignment of the eye and tracking systems are not necessary. Although the operating time is short, this system requires a high energy to achieve the required ablation and delivers a greater acoustic shock wave to the cornea. The high-output energy requirement results in a more frequent maintenance of the optical components and an increase in the overall running cost. Limited ablation patterns are available and a higher incidence of central islands has also been reported with the wide field ablation system. The Summit: Apex plus, Omnimed, Excimed, VISX: Star, Model B, Twenty/Twenty B, Coherent-Schwind Keratom and the Chiron-Technolas Keracor 116 are examples of this class of excimer lasers.

Scanning Slit Ablation

Scanning slit ablation is the second generation photorefractive delivery system. It employs a rectangular slit-shaped beam of light that scans across an aperture within the path of the beam and uniformly removes tissue with several successive pulses of laser. The amount of tissue removed varies depending on the amount of overlap between the pulses.

The scanning slit ablation requires a lower pulse energy output and ensures an excellent beam uniformity and homogeneity because of the small area being ablated with each pulse. The small area ablation produces a smoother ablative surface and also reduces the complication of central islands. No optic zone limitations are present. However the ablation takes a longer time to complete and requires a complex scanning system with eye tracking facilities. The Nidek EC-5000 (Fig. 6.1) and Meditec MEL 60 use this technology.

Flying (Scanning) Spot Ablation

This is the latest development in laser delivery systems. The third generation flying spot laser performs scanning in multiple directions to remove a uniform

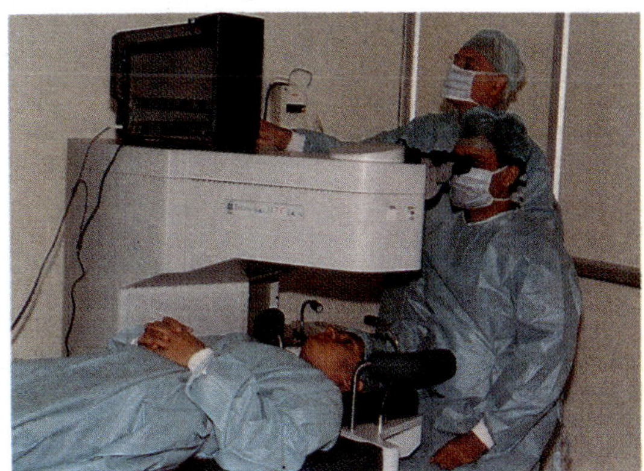

Fig. 6.1: Nidek EC 5000 excimer laser machine

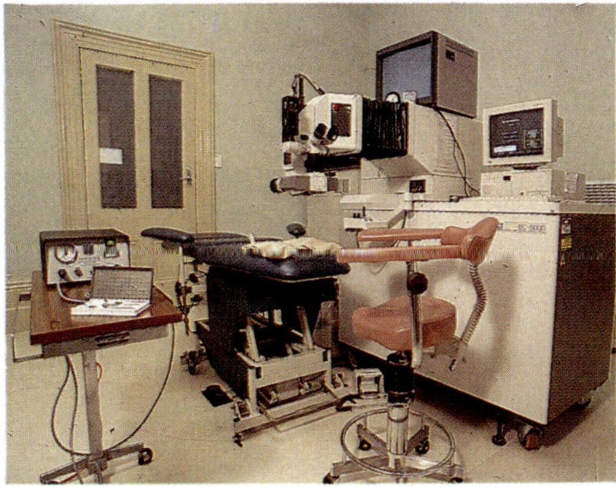

Fig. 6.2: Chiron Technolas 217 excimer laser workstation

layer of corneal tissue. It allows for a custom designed ablation and uses the lowest energy output. The cost of maintenance and the number of optics in the machine are also reduced. Large zone ablations with complex ablation patterns (including hyperopia) are possible. The main disadvantage is that it requires the longest operating time and therefore precise eye tracking systems are required. A high repetition rate is necessary and since it is relatively a new technology, the algorithms have still not been perfected. The Novatec Light blade (non excimer solid state laser), Laser Sight Compak 200, Kera Technology ISO beam and the Chiron Technolas Keracor 117 and 217 (Fig. 6.2) are examples of the machines which use the flying spot technology.

Seven

Surgical Technique

Once the preoperative assessment has been completed, the patient is scheduled for surgery. On the day of the surgery, the surgeon must examine each patient again, rule out ocular infection and verify the various refractive measurements. The patient is instructed to wash his or her face and eyelids with soap and water. The two most important parameters to be checked are the corneal pachymetry and the size of the pupil in scotopic conditions, as these two factors determine the amount of ablation possible and the size of the optic zone. Generally a residual stromal thickness of 250 microns is desirable and the amount of ablation to be done can be calculated by using the Munnerlyn formula : $T = (DH^2)/3$, where T is the thickness of the stromal corneal tissue ablation in microns, D is the power in dioptres, and H is the diameter of the optic zone in millimetres. The scotopic pupillary size determines the problems the patient is likely to face during night vision, and therefore it needs to be taken into consideration while feeding the data pertaining to the diameter of the ablation zone. The surgeon must ensure that the consent form has been read by the patient and signed. The patient should be instructed to look into the fixation light, not to squeeze the eyelids and not to bring his or her hands onto the operative field. The feeling of pressure when the suction ring is placed on the eye is very uncomfortable for some patients and the patient needs to be reassured about the same.

Although there may be some individual variations in the LASIK technique, most of the surgical steps of LASIK are common to all individual techniques. These are as follows:

Preparation of the Operating Room

An optimal operating room environment and the practice of an aseptic surgical technique are of extreme importance for LASIK. The operation theatre should have a particle-free environment, have a temperature maintained between 15 and 25 degree celsius, and a humidity level of less than 50 per cent. This is important because any change in the temperature or the humidity, alters the fluence of the laser and the standard ablation rates. A filtration unit is a must and should be functional a few hours prior to starting the laser. An uninterruptable power supply should be ensured. The excimer laser machine requires a round the clock air-conditioning unit. It is mandatory that all laser equipments, electrical connections and surgical instruments be checked before starting the surgery. It is important to ensure that the gas level is adequate in the excimer laser machine and the microkeratome is functioning properly.

Instruments

The surgeon should check the laser machine (Fig. 7.1), the eye tracking system (Fig. 7.2), the foot switches (Fig. 7.3), the assembled head of the microkeratome (Fig. 7.4), and the console for power supply (Fig. 7.5). A new blade should be used (Fig. 7.6), engaged with the pin (Fig. 7.7), inserted into the head of the

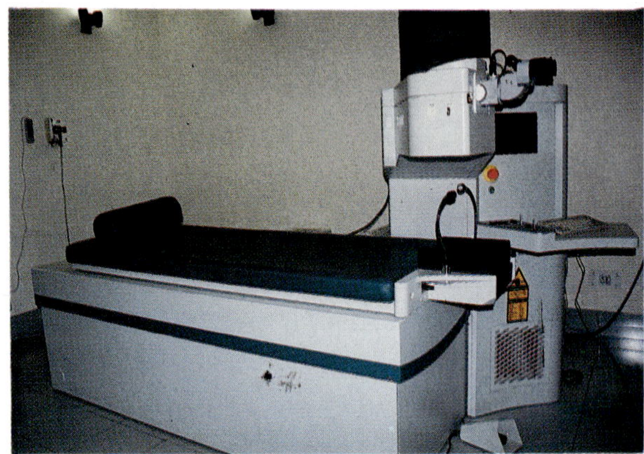

Fig. 7.1: Chiron Technolas 217 excimer laser workstation

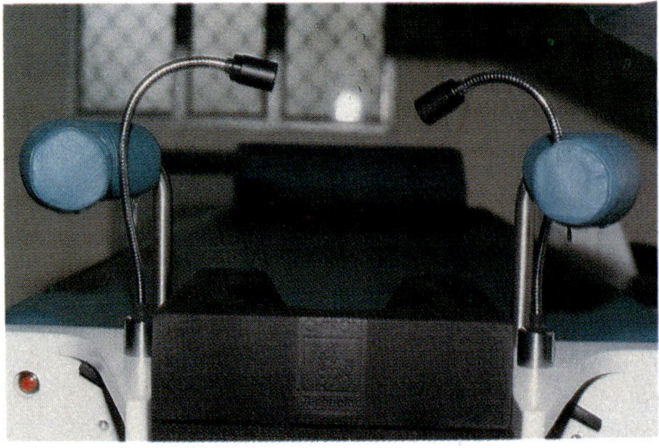

Fig. 7.2: Head rest for the patient with the two eye trackers

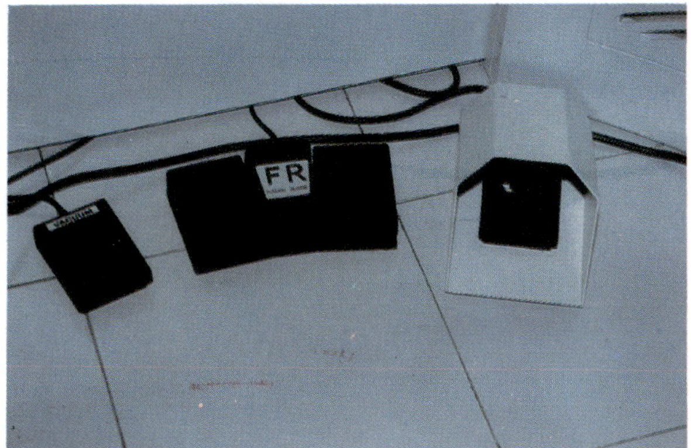

Fig. 7.3: Footswitches for suction (left), movement of the microkeratome (middle) and laser delivery (right)

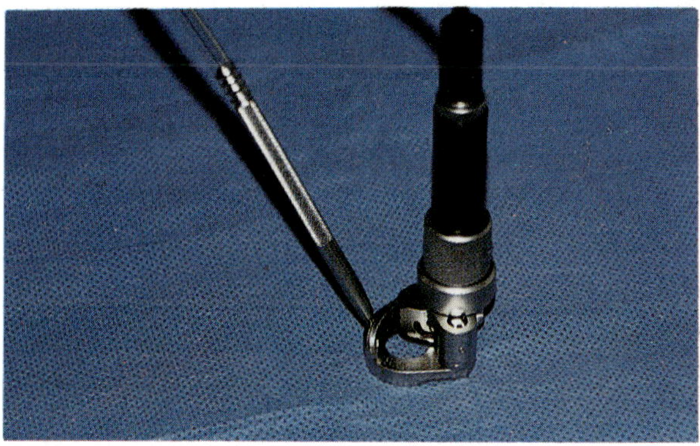

Fig. 7.4: Hansatome microkeratome attached to the suction ring

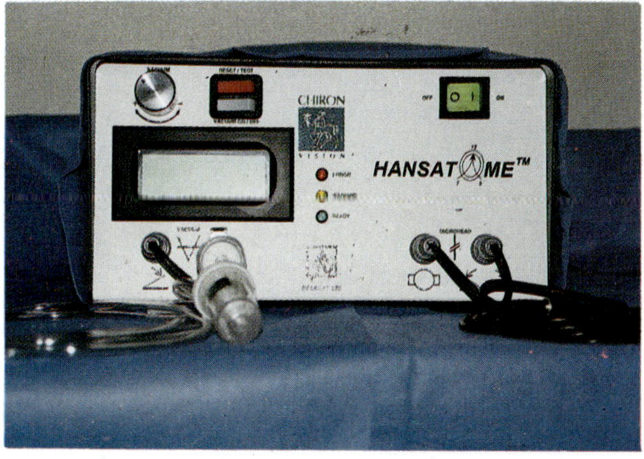

Fig. 7.5: Power supply unit of the Hansatome

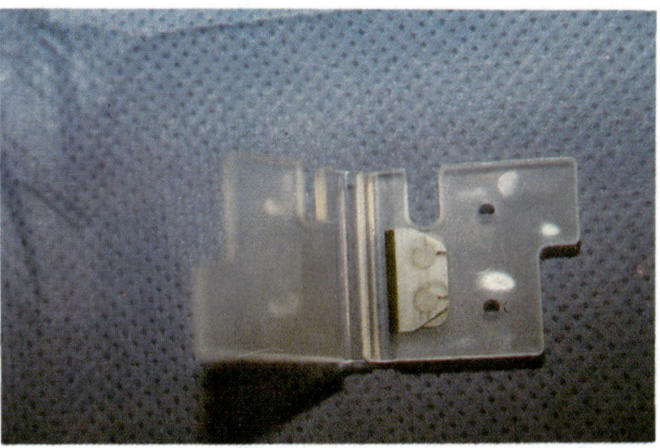

Fig. 7.6: Sterile blade of the Hansatome in a plastic case

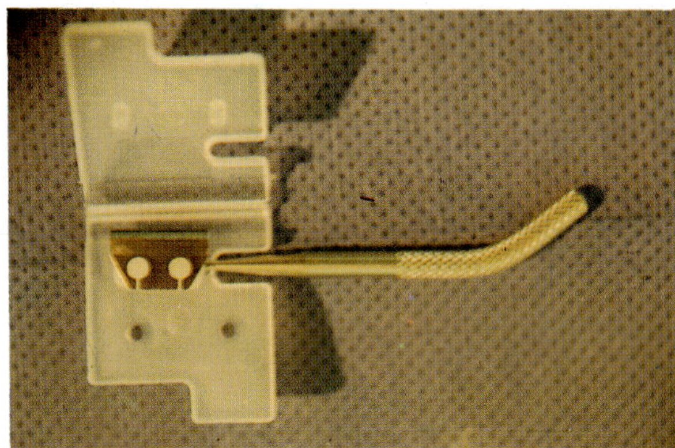

Fig. 7.7: Blade handling pin engaging the blade

microkeratome (Fig. 7.8) and checked again (Fig. 7.9). The suction rings (Fig. 7.10) microkeratome heads (Fig. 7.11) and the eye adapter (Fig. 7.12) should be examined.

The instrument tray of the microkeratome should be kept ready (Fig. 7.13). Other instruments required for LASIK surgery include: lid speculum (Fig. 7.14), suction speculum (Fig. 7.15), Merocal sponges (Fig. 7.16), steridrape (Fig. 7.17), corneal markers (Fig. 7.18), corneal spatula (Fig. 7.19), flap protector (Fig. 7.20), tonometer (Fig. 7.21), temperature and humidity gauge (Fig. 7.22) and the trolley for arranging all these instruments (Fig. 7.23).

Surgeon Preparation

The same surgical preparation is followed as for an intraocular procedure by scrubbing, wearing of surgical cap and mask, and putting on powder-free gloves which need to be changed after every case.

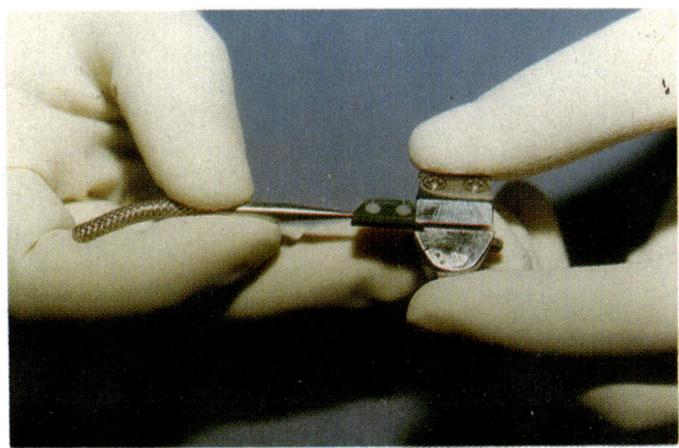

Fig. 7.8: Blade being inserted into the head of the Hansatome

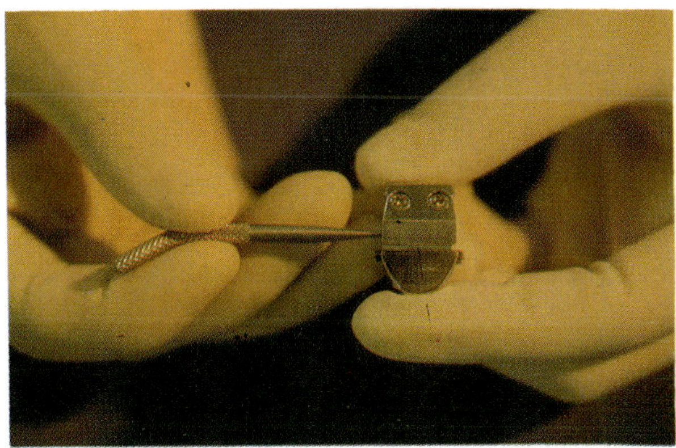

Fig. 7.9: Correction position of the blade after
insertion into the microkeratome head

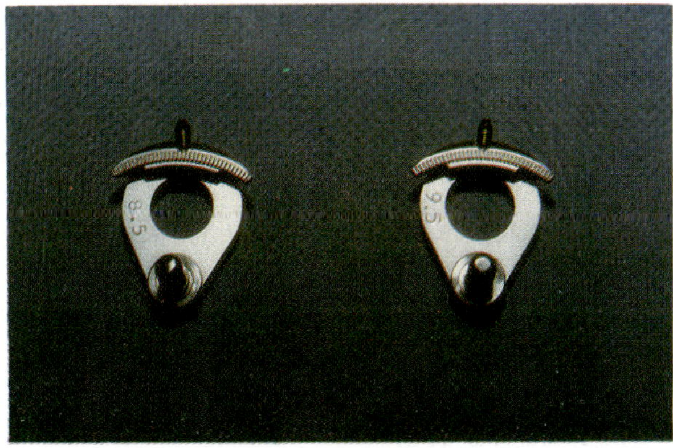

Fig. 7.10: 8.5 cm and 9.5 cm diameter suction rings
for use with the Hansatome

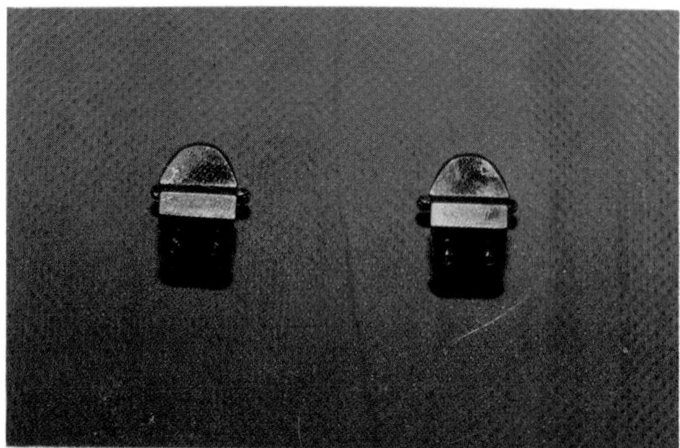

Fig. 7.11: Two heads of the Hansatome for creating a
160 microns and 180 microns depth flap

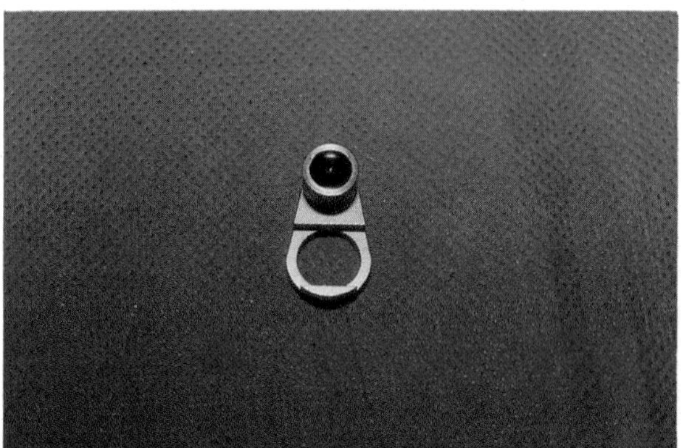

Fig. 7.12: The eye adapter for using the Hansatome on the right/left eye

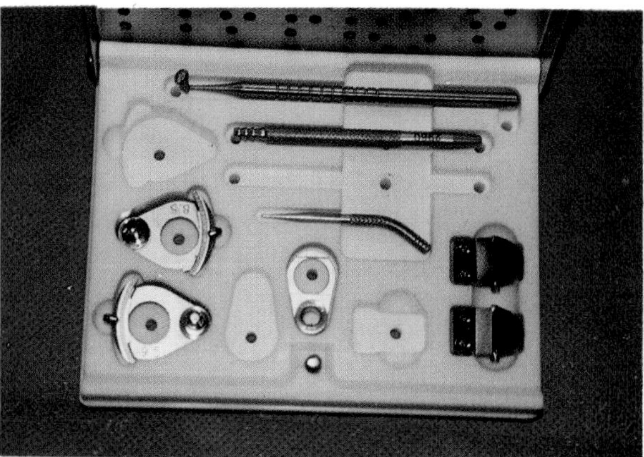

Fig. 7.13: Instrument tray of the Hansatome with the suction rings, eye adapter,
microkeratome heads, blade handling pin, suction ring handle and corneal marker

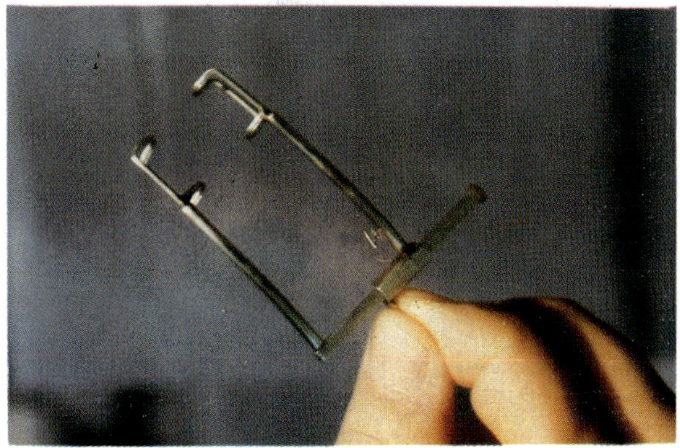

Fig. 7.14: Adjustable lid speculum

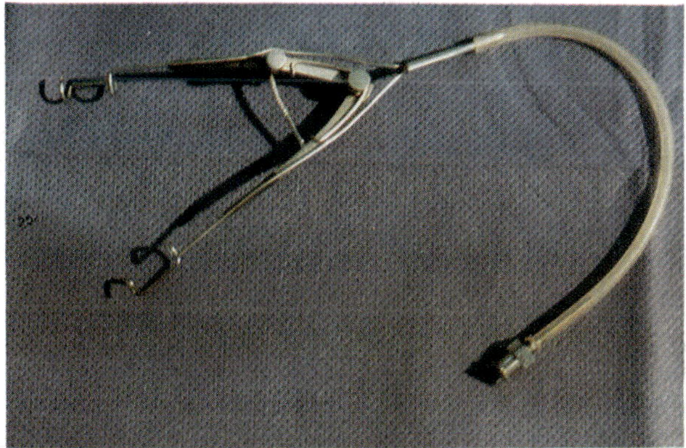

Fig. 7.15: Suction speculum

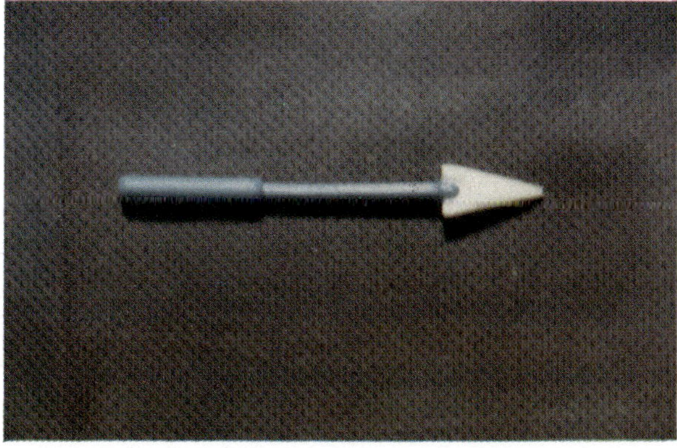

Fig. 7.16: Merocel sponge

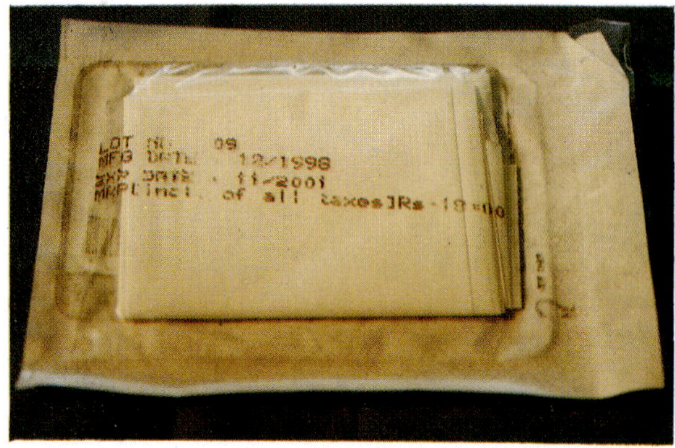

Fig. 7.17: Steridrape

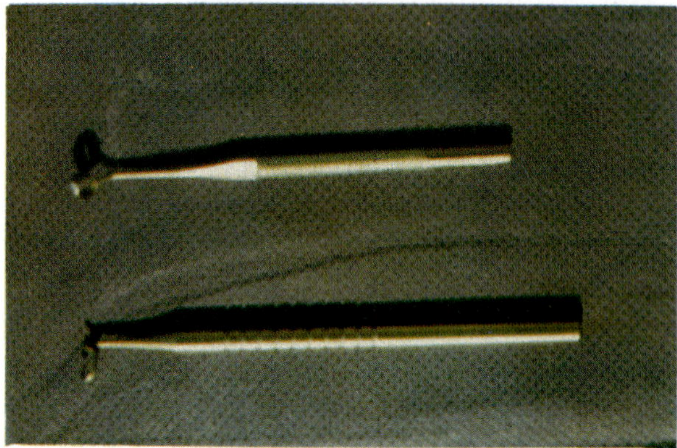

Fig. 7.18: Corneal markers

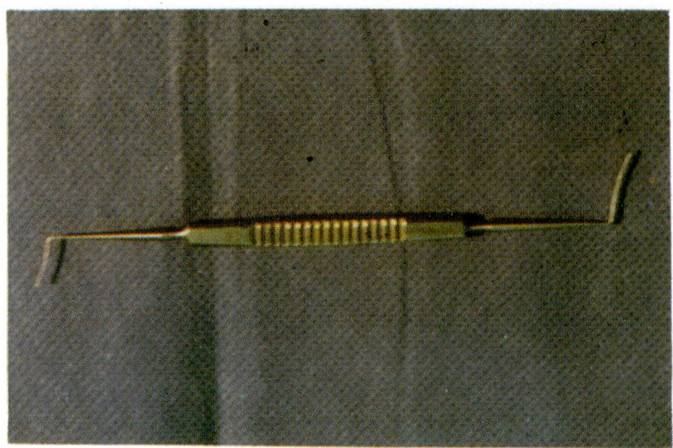

Fig. 7.19: Spatula for lifting the corneal flap

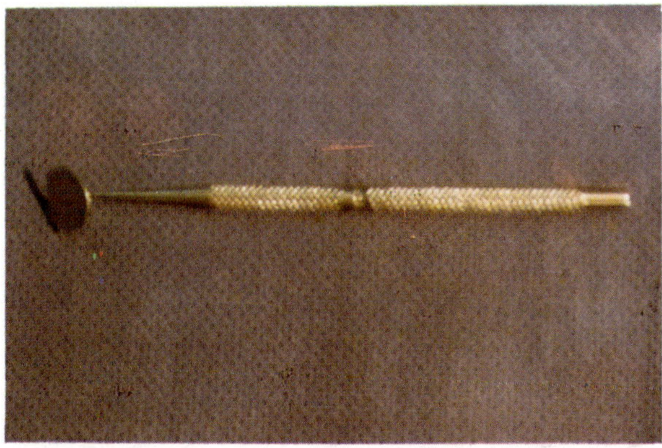

Fig. 7.20: Flap protection for covering the hinge of the flap during laser ablation

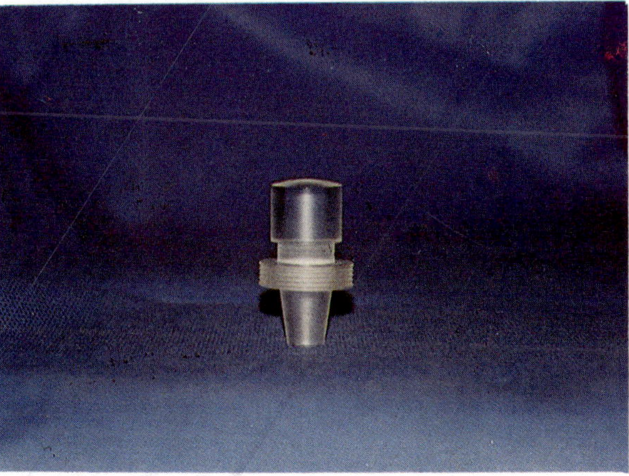

Fig. 7.21: Barraquer tonometer

Patient Preparation

Some surgeons prefer to sedate the patient pre-operatively with an oral sedative, such as diazepam, half an hour or so before the commencement of LASIK surgery. Most surgeons however find that this is not necessary. The patient's face and eyelids are cleaned with soap and water, dried and then the eye to be operated is cleaned with 5% povidone-iodine solution. A broad-spectrum antibiotic (0.3% ciprofloxacin) or 0.5% povidone-iodine drops are instilled into the conjunctival fornix one hour prior to the surgery. The patient is asked to wear a cap while in the operating room. The patient's head must be placed parallel to the floor and the chin and the forehead should be at the same level. It is important to ensure that the patient's cornea is perpendicular to the laser beam (Fig. 7.24), especially

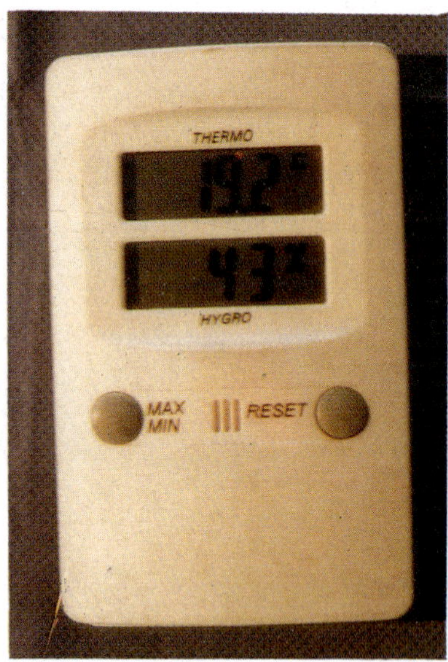

Fig. 7.22: Instrument for monitoring the temperature and humidity of the operating room

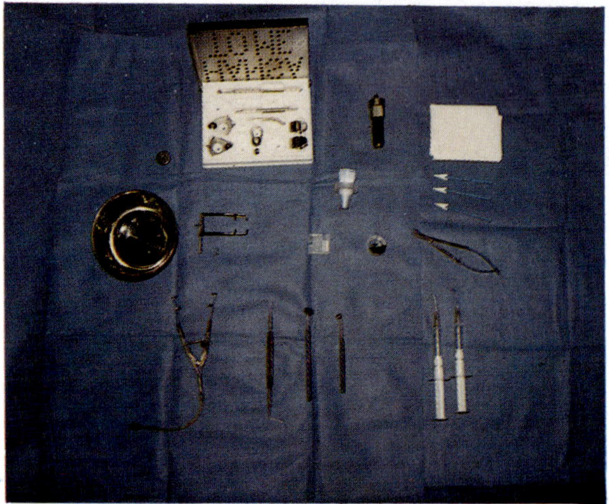

Fig. 7.23: Instrument trolley for LASIK

for astigmatic ablations. The patient is instructed to look at the fixation light and the fellow eye is covered by a plastic shield. The patient should wear a tag mentioning his or her name, clinic reference number and the refractive error, so that the surgeon can cross-check the particulars of the patient before proceeding ahead with the surgery.

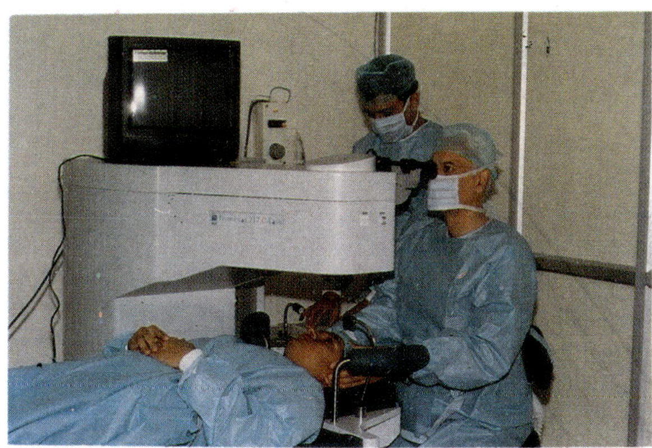

Fig. 7.24: Correct positioning of the patient with the cornea
perpendicular to the aiming beam of the laser

Topical anaesthetic drops [4% lidocaine or 0.5% proparacaine] are instilled into the eye 5 to 10 minutes prior to surgery and just before inserting the speculum.

The patient is then positioned under the laser's microscope. A fenestrated sterile plastic drape is placed with the eyes wide open, so that eyelashes do not enter in the operative field. Surgical tape may also be used to hold the lashes out of the way. The cornea is exposed by separating the eyelids with a (Fig. 7.25) speculum. For an extremely anxious patient, some surgeons prefer to induce eyelid akinesia using a facial nerve block. Additional irrigation and removal of any secretions with a sponge may be required after insertion of the speculum

Corneal Marking

To ensure correct and exact replacement of the corneal flap at the end of LASIK surgery, the peripheral cornea is marked just prior to surgery (Fig. 7.26). A variety of different markers have been developed for this purpose. The marker is stained with methylene blue or gentian violet and is applied firmly to the dry cornea. A minimal quantity of gentian violet is to be used because it is toxic to the epithelium.

It is preferable to use a central 8 mm ring marker, followed by three, 3 mm ring marks placed superiorly, temporally and inferiorly. Although this may look somewhat combersome, it takes little extra time and allows for the more precise realignment of the corneal flap after its replacement. The importance of corneal marking is especially evident in case of a free cap, where the marks provide the only clue to a proper alignment.

Application of Suction Ring

After marking the cornea, the pneumatic fixation ring is applied to the eyeball and the vacuum is activated (Fig. 7.27). The patient is informed of a pressure

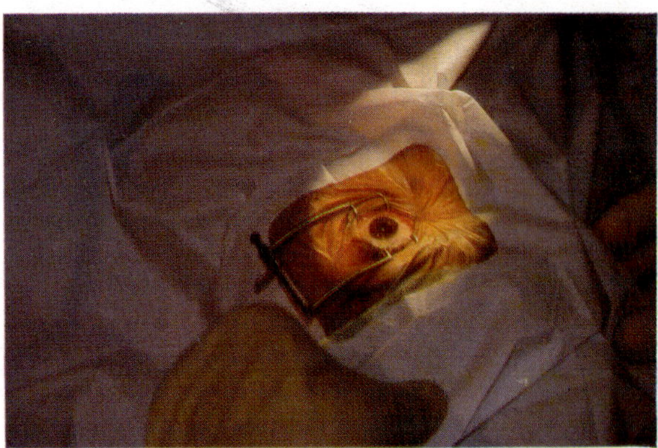

Fig. 7.25: Application of the steridrape and lid speculum to obtain maximal exposure of the eyeball

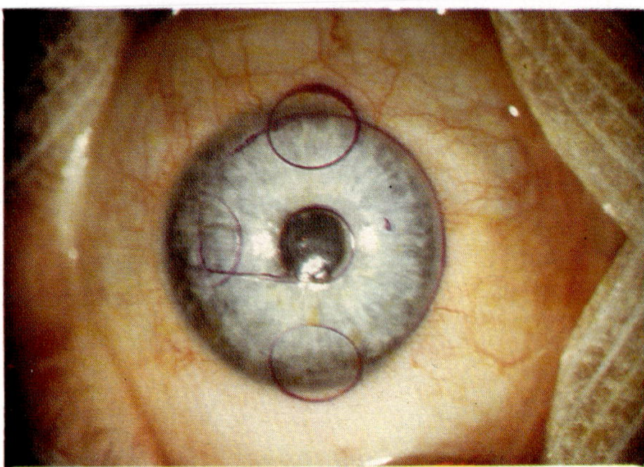

Fig. 7.26: Marking of the cornea with gentian violet

sensation and the blurring of vision during this procedure. After the suction ring has been placed, a drop of 0.5% proparacaine or distilled water (Fig. 7.28) can be put on the cornea before the microkeratome is placed. One should avoid using a salt solution (BSS, normal saline, Ringer lactate) as the salt crystals can accumulate on the suction ring track and obstruct the movement of the microkeratome. While using the Hansatome, we use the 9.5 mm suction ring if the corneal diameter is more than 10.5 mm and the 8.5 mm ring if it is less than 10.5 mm.

Tonometry

A good suction and a high intraocular pressure (IOP) are the most important prerequisites for the cut with the microkeratome. It is therefore important to check the IOP with a tonometer (such as the Barraquer's tonometer). The IOP should be more than 65 mm Hg before one can proceed with the pass of the

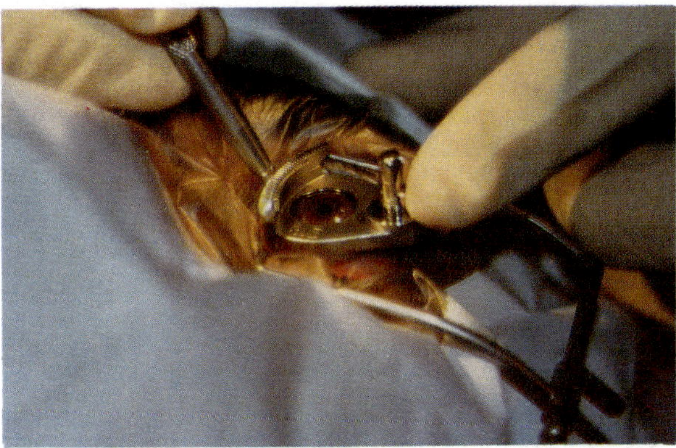

Fig. 7.27: Application of the suction ring on to the eyeball

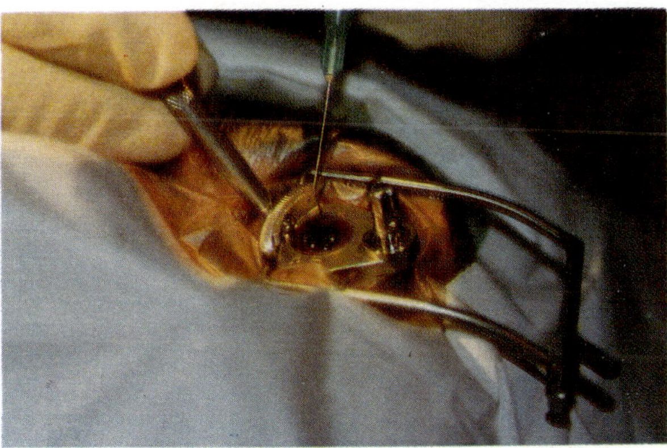

Fig. 7.28: Irrigation of the cornea with distilled water after placing the suction ring

microkeratome. While using the Barraquer's tonometer (Fig. 7.29), the applanation area should be well within the circular mire inscribed on the tonometer as this indicates an IOP of more than 65 mm Hg (Fig. 7.30). If the IOP is not raised sufficiently, it can cause problems during the cutting of the cornea and may create a flap that is suboptimal in terms of diameter, thickness and the quality of the cut surface. Digital tonometry should not be a criteria for assessing the adequacy of the IOP, as it is often inaccurate.

Creation of Corneal Flap

Performance of the cut to create a corneal flap is the most delicate and important step of the LASIK procedure. Most surgeons prefer a flap of 180 μm thickness (a thicker flap is easier to handle) and with a diameter of 8.5 mm or more. A large diameter flap is desirable for hyperopic LASIK.

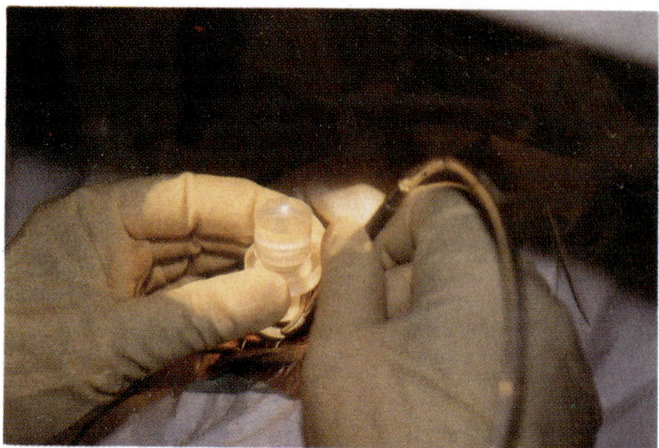

Fig. 7.29: Checking the IOP with the Barraquer tonometer

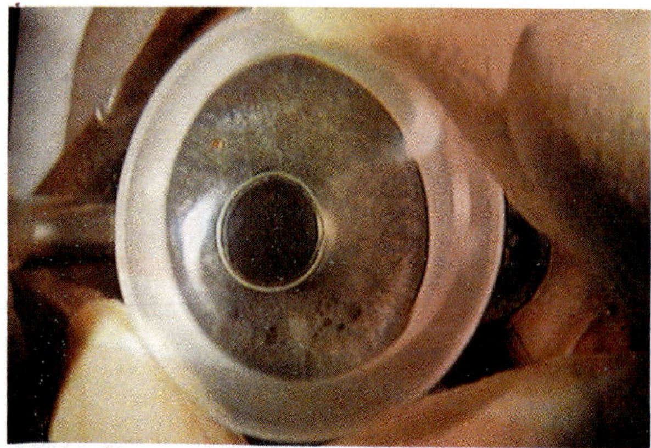

Fig. 7.30: Central mire just inside the circular mark etched
on the Barraquer tonometer, indicating an IOP of more than 65 mm Hg

Before applying microkeratome to the cornea, it is mandatory that all the components are thoroughly checked and assembled properly. A disposable preassembled microkeratome also needs to be thoroughly checked and tested. The surgeon has to ascertain that microkeratome is moving smoothly over the entire track by performing a complete forward and reverse pass. The instruments should be carefully observed under the microscope and it is important to look for any debris on the microkeratome head or the suction ring.

After the microkeratome is applied to the cornea (Fig. 7.31), the first part of foot pedal (F-forward switch) is activated to advance the microkeratome along the suction ring, up to the stop device. After the completion of the initial cut, the second part of foot pedal (R- reverse switch) is activated to reverse the microkeratome to its original position. After the completion of the cut, the vacuum of the

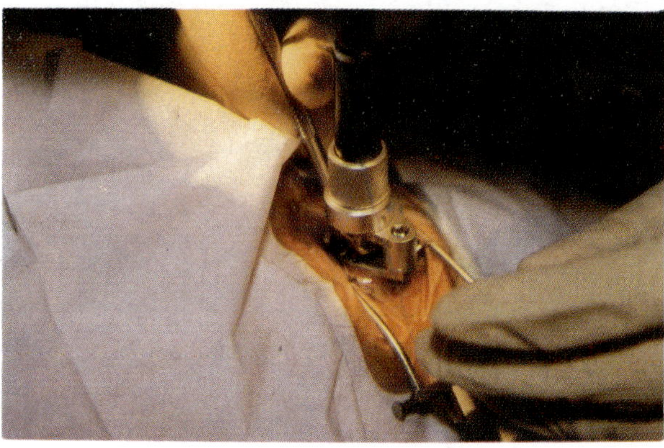

Fig. 7.31: Application of the Hansatome on to the suction ring

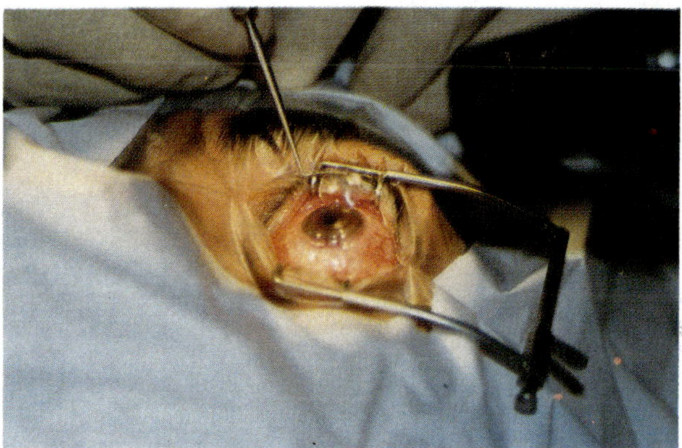

Fig. 7.32: Insertion of the spatula under the corneal flap

suction ring is released and microkeratome is disengaged. The flap thus created is flipped over to the nasal or superior perilimbal conjunctival surface using a blunt spatula (Figs 7.32 to 7.33) or a forceps. The exposed corneal stroma is wiped dry with a Merocel sponge. Any flap related complications are looked for before proceeding on with the laser. The assistant can exert a downward pressure on the speculum during the movement of the microkeratome. This helps to ensure a good exposure, causes a slight proptosis of the globe and irons out any folds in the conjunctiva which can block the suction ports in the suction ring.

Excimer Laser Ablation

The laser is preprogrammed to perform a corneal stromal ablation appropriate for the magnitude and type of the refractive error. Some lasers use an eye-tracking system to deal with the problem of decentration caused by the eye movements.

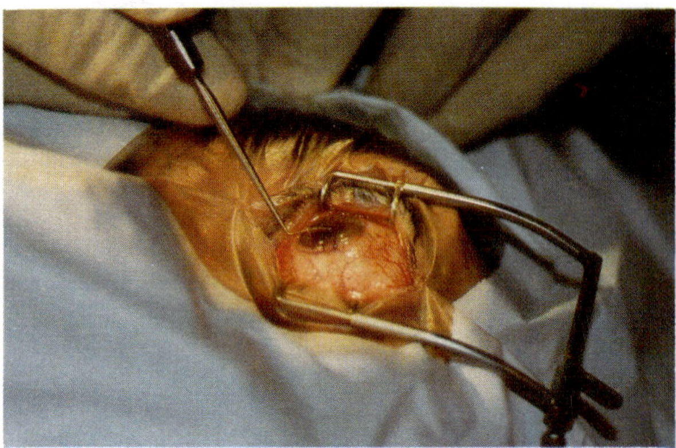

Fig. 7.33: Lifting up the flap with the spatula

However, it is advisable that the centration of the patient's eye is checked again after the creation of the flap and the patient be repeatedly directed to look at the fixation light. The coaxial illumination of the microscope should be decreased to minimise glare and allow a good patient fixation. If during the cut, the patient's eye and head have moved from the original position, this should be corrected and the cornea should be perpendicular to the laser beam.

The cornea should not be excessively wet or dry during the ablation as it may lead to ablation of less or more tissue than intended. Also care must be taken during the ablation, to protect the hinge of the flap. This can be done by retracting the flap as much as possible (Fig. 7.34) or by shielding the hinge with a specially designed spatula or a damp Merocel sponge.

The fluence of the laser should be checked after each case or after 10,000 laser shots.

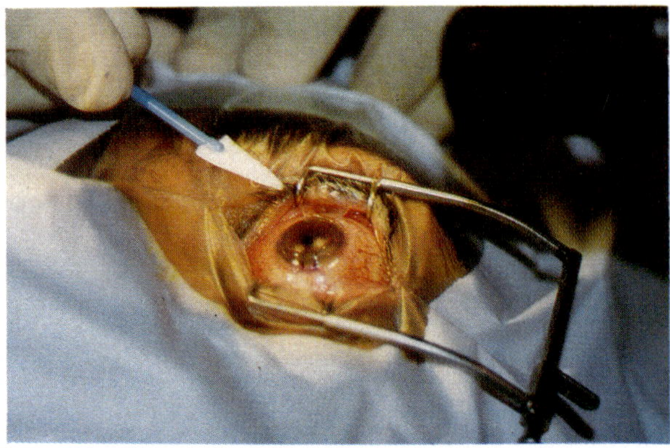

Fig. 7.34: Laser ablation of the stromal bed with the flap resting
on the steridrape at the upper lid margin

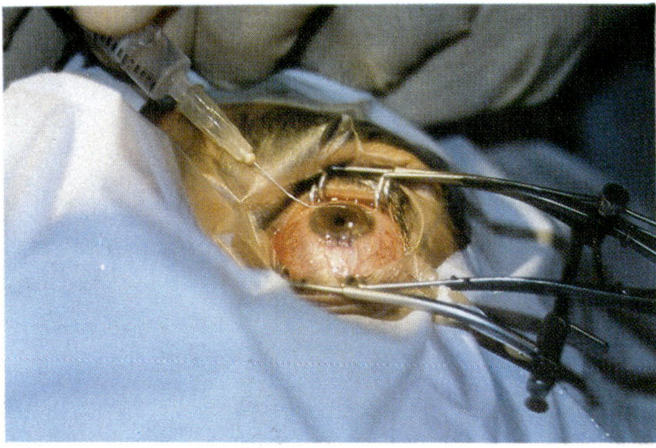

Fig. 7.35: Repositioning of the flap and irrigation of the undersurface of the flap

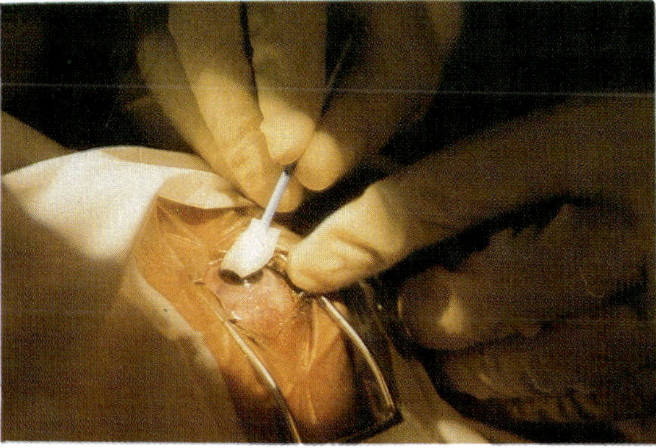

Fig. 7.36: Gentle massage of flap downward from the hinge with a wet Merocel sponge

Replacement of the Flap

After the completion of excimer laser ablation, a drop or two of distilled water is placed on the stromal surface, the flap is reposited back immediately and the stromal bed is irrigated under the flap to remove any debris from the interface (Fig. 7.35). Excess of fluid is removed by gently wiping the flap away from the hinge with a moistened Merocel sponge (Fig. 7.36) and the alignment of the flap is confirmed using the preplaced reference marks. During alignment, the centre of the flap is kept moist and the peripheral gutter is dried to facilitate adhesion of the flap to the stromal bed. After 2 to 3 minutes, the peripheral cornea is depressed and the translation of the resultant striae onto the flap (striae test) is taken as evidence of optimal adhesion. The speculum and drapes are carefully removed without touching the cornea and the patient is asked to gently close the eyelids.

The correct re-positioning of the flap is again confirmed, an antibiotic eyedrop is instilled and a clear plastic shield is applied to the eye. In addition to protecting the eye the transparent plastic shield allows the patient to see and prevents the patient from rubbing the eye, an important precaution in the postoperative period. Some surgeons prefer to use a bandage contact lens to protect the flap.

The following factors help to secure the the flap back into position: capillary attraction of the tissues, endothelial pump action, migration of epithelium over the cut edges and scarring along the cut edge of Bowman's membrane.

Eight

Postoperative Management

Most surgeons prefer to examine their patients on the slit lamp within an hour or so after the surgery, to check for the correct placement and adhesion of the flap. This early examination allows for rectification of any folds or displacement of the flap and removal of interface debris, if significant. On the day of the surgery the patient is instructed to go home and sleep for a few hours, as lid closure facilitates rapid epithelialisation of the perpheral gutter created by the lamellar keratectomy. It is important to counsel the patients with regards to the vision and the discomfort after the surgery. Mild pain and foreign body sensation may persist up to 24 hours and the vision may be blurred up to 48 hours. The patients should be warned about subconjunctival haemorrhages, which may be a common occurrence after LASIK. In addition the patient should be explained about the variability of the response between the two eyes.

Subsequent postoperative examinations are scheduled at 24 hours, 1 week, 1, 3, 6 and 12 months. At each follow-up visit, a complete ophthalmic examination is conducted, including a record of the uncorrected and best corrected visual acuity, refraction, slit-lamp biomicroscopy and videokeratography. The change in contrast sensitivity and glare should also to be noted.

The patient must be instructed not to rub his or her eye for 2 weeks, avoid swimming for 2 weeks and use sunglasses during the day and a plastic shield at night. Normal work schedule and everyday activities can be resumed on the day after the operation. All activities that can cause trauma to the eye should be avoided and the patient should be informed that driving may be difficult due to fluctuations in visual acuity in the first postoperative week. If there is pain, redness and marked blurring of vision at any time during the postoperative period, the patient should be asked to report immediately to the treating doctor, as this may signify an infection or a flap dislocation.

Postoperative prophylactic antibiotic drops are used four times a day for 7 days. Broad-spectrum antibiotics such as chloramphenicol, tobramycin and ciprofloxacin should be used. Some surgeons use steroid eyedrops such as fluorometholone (FML) in the first week or so after LASIK, but many surgeons prefer to use non-steroidal anti-inflammatory drugs (NSAIDs) such as diclofenac or ketorolac, for the first week. An antibiotic-steroid combination is also a popular option. In addition, wetting agents should be used to maintain tear film stability during the early postoperative period. Some patients may require oral analgesics on the day of the surgery. If the patient experiences disabling problems with night vision, one drop of dilute pilocarpine may be required in the evening (0.125% or 0.25%).

Postoperative Examination Protocol

The following details are to be noted in the follow-up examinations done at one hour after the surgery, 24 hours, 7 days, 1 month, 3 months and 6 months after the surgery. The examination done one hour and 24 hours after the surgery is the most crucial one for detection of flap-related complications.

One hour — The most important parameter to be evaluated is the adherence of the flap. A careful slit-lamp examination should be performed to ascertain that the entire flap is well apposed. The surgeon should also look for any folds and wrinkles in the flap and shifting or dislodgement of the flap. Interface debris (especially metal fillings, fibres or epithelial tags) under the flap should be ruled out. If any of the above mentioned abnormalities are present, the surgeon needs to take immediate corrective steps by relifting the flap, irrigating the stromal bed and the interface and repositing the flap back.

Twenty-four hours — The examination on the first postoperative day is important to ensure that re-epithelialisation is complete over the edges of the flap. Shifting or dislodgement of the flap, flap wrinkling, folding, interface debris, and any evidence of postoperative keratitis (sterile/infectious) needs to be examined at this stage. The uncorrected visual acuity (UCVA) should also be recorded.

The examination conducted 1 week after the surgery and then at subsequent follow-ups should include a thorough evaluation of the following parameters: Uucorrected and best corrected visual acuity, refraction and determination of the residual refractive error, keratometry, pachymetry, corneal topography, contrast sensitivity, glare and corneal endothelial count. A clinical photograph of the flap should be taken and a diagram depicting any flap abnormality should be entered in the file of the patient for future reference.

Nine

LASIK Complications and Management

In comparison to other techniques of refractive surgery including photorefractive keratectomy, LASIK is a relatively complex surgical procedure. Each step of LASIK surgery demands meticulous attention and surgical skill of a high order. Any deviation from prescribed surgical protocol can lead to potentially disastrous complications.

The complications of LASIK may be related to problems with the microkeratome, the laser ablation, the size or shape of the eye, or to the healing process. The various complications may be divided into three categories: preoperative, intraoperative and postoperative.

PREOPERATIVE COMPLICATIONS

Anaesthesia

Excess application of topical anaesthesia can be toxic to the epithelium and may cause epithelial oedema and sloughing.

Drape and Speculum

Corneal abrasions and epithelial defects can occur while inserting the speculum and applying or removing the drape. These can delay visual recovery and interfere in the microkeratome cut.

Corneal Marking

The gentian violet dye used for marking the cornea can produce toxic changes in the corneal epithelium and aggressive indentation used to create the mark can induce irregularities on the corneal surface.

Inadequate Exposure

Variations in the normal orbital anatomy such as deep set eyes, small palpebral fissure or changes induced by orbital or lid trauma may lead to an inadequate exposure. A poor draping technique or a poor choice of the eye speculum may also contribute to this problem. If the exposure is not adequate, there can be difficulty in placing the suction ring, failure to achieve adequate suction and an incomplete microkeratome pass due to interference from the drape or the speculum. A strong spring or locking speculum should be used to achieve maximal exposure and the assistant should apply downward pressure on the speculum during the pass of the microkeratome. A lateral canthotomy may be necessary in some cases.

Inadequate Suction

Inadequate exposure, a small corneal diameter, microkeratome malfunction and manipulations of the suction ring or the speculum can be the various causes of an inadequate suction. This can lead to a thin flap or a buttonhole. The best way to prevent this complication is to measure the intraocular pressure (IOP) with the Barraquer's tonometer before proceeding with the microkeratome pass, to ensure that suction is adequate. The exposure should be optimal and the suction ring should be firmly pressed against the globe when the suction is turned on.

INTRAOPERATIVE COMPLICATIONS

Microkeratome-related Complications

The microkeratome is a complex device and only a well-trained and skilled ophthalmic surgeon who has bimanual dexterity and gives full attention to detail can successfully use it. It is imperative that full adherence to the manufacturer's recommendations regarding a particular microkeratome is followed. A defective microkeratome or its incorrect use may cause the following complications in the patient's eye.

Corneal Perforation

A corneal perforation during the corneal cut is a result of improper seating of thickness plate or failure to install it at all. The microkeratome blade without the restraint of the thickness plate, can perforate the cornea during the pass and the intraocular contents, including lens and vitreous can be expulsed, as during the surgery the IOP is kept very high [>60 mm Hg]. This complication does not occur with microkeratomes that have a preassembled fixed thickness plate. It is also important to rule out corneal ectatic disorders which are an absolute contraindication to a lamellar corneal cut, as is performed in LASIK.

Management

If corneal perforation occurs, the suction should be turned off immediately and the procedure terminated. The tissues should be repaired, usually under general anaesthesia. Depending on the severity of the complication, repair may include suturing of the cornea, reconstruction of the anterior chamber or a lensectomy/vitrectomy.

Incomplete Flap

If a microkeratome stops in the middle of a pass and does not complete its travel across the cornea, an incomplete cut results, producing an incomplete flap. The various factors that can cause an incomplete flap include loss of the motor power, blockage of the foot pedal or the microkeratome, inadvertent pressure on the foot pedal and premature release of suction by the surgeon, insufficient suction, interference by the lid or the speculum and presence of any debris along the microkeratome track. Eyes with scleral buckling surgery and dense conjunctival scarring are at high risk of not being able to develop a sufficient suction and IOP elevation for the creation of a good flap with the microkeratome. It is important to run the microkeratome through a complete cycle prior to use in each eye of a patient, to ensure proper functioning.

Management

If the microkeratome stops in the initial stages of a cut (within central 6-7 mm zone), the LASIK surgery should be stopped and the microkeratome is reversed. The suction ring should be removed and the partial flap replaced. Surgery can be attempted again three months later and at this time it is better to use the 180 µm plate. If the microkeratome has performed a major portion of the cut before stopping and there is an adequate space for laser ablation, one may proceed with the laser, keeping a smaller optic zone and protecting the hinge of the flap. If the keratectomy has proceeded beyond the optic zone before the malfunction, then one can consider the manual completion of the lamellar dissection, although most surgeons warn against doing this.

Thin Flap

Sometimes the flap that is created is thin and irregular in thickness (Fig. 9.1). These flaps are liable to be torn easily and there may be a full thickness *buttonhole* (Figs 9.2 and 9.3) in the flap. Inadequate suction or loss of suction during the movement of microkeratome across the cornea is a major cause of this complication. Steep corneas may buckle under the foot plate of the microkeratome and lead to the creation of a central buttonhole. Conjunctival chemosis and oedema caused by repeated applications of the suction ring to achieve optimal corneal centration, is another factor responsible for loss of suction during the cut. Alterations in the speed of advancement of the keratome along the track, insufficient elevation of the IOP, a small lid fissure and uncontrolled blinking by the patient are other risk factors responsible for the occurrence of such a

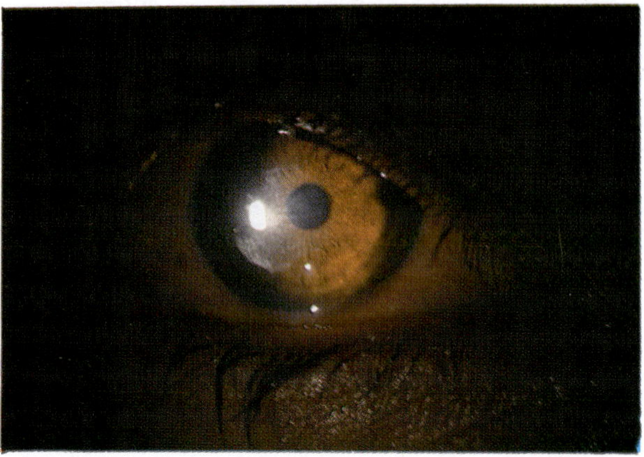

Fig. 9.1: Postoperative scarring in an eye with a thin and irregular flap

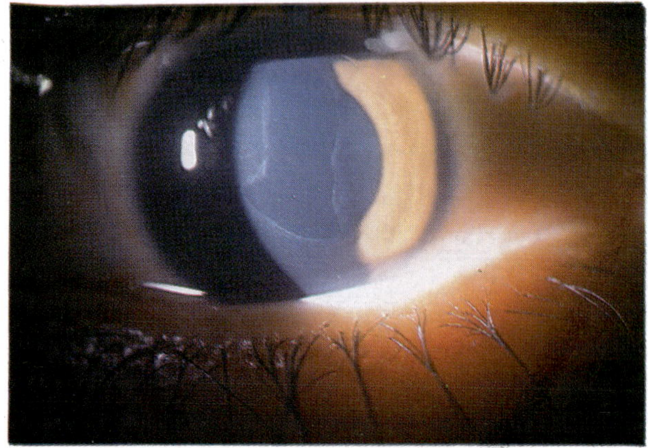

Fig. 9.2: Central buttonhole in the flap

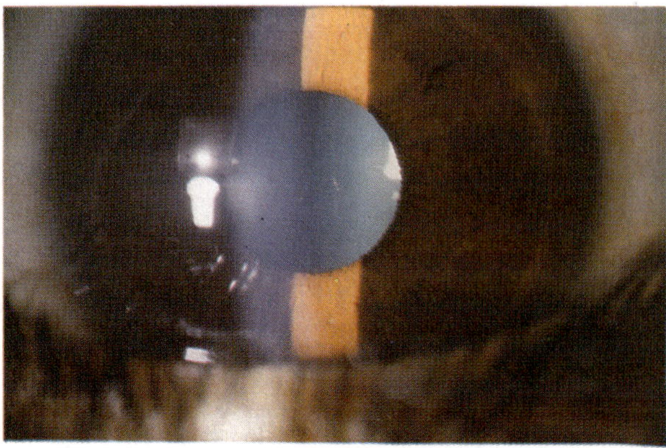

Fig. 9.3: Linear scar caused by a previous buttonhole in the flap

complication. There is an increased risk of irregular astigmatism and epithelial ingrowth with the creation of thin and irregular flaps.

Management

If the flap is irregular it should be returned to the original position without laser treatment. The flap should be properly inspected and the adherence verified. The operation should be postponed for three months and then repeated with a deeper cut. Patients with steep corneas (> 46 D) should be warned about the occurrence of this complication and deeper depth plate used in such eyes.

Free Cap

Failure to obtain a hinge while completing the creation of the flap can occur if the stop mechanism of the microkeratome has not been fitted properly. Surgery on a large and very flat (< 41 D) cornea can also lead to free caps.

Management

If a free cap is made, it is best to carefully remove it from the microkeratome head and place in an antidesiccation chamber with the epithelial side down, on a drop of balanced salt solution (BSS). The laser treatment is performed as usual and then the flap is carefully replaced using the reference marks to guide its relocation. Free flaps usually sit well if carefully handled and the waiting time after cap replacement should be increased to 5 minutes to ensure an adequate adherence. Rarely do they need to be sutured with a 10/0 nylon suture.

Bleeding from Limbal Vessels

In addition to the above mentioned complications, bleeding from limbal vessels which have been cut during the pass of the microkeratome, is a common problem while performing LASIK and can lead to corneal blood staining (Fig. 9.4). This especially occurs if a large foot plate diameter is used in a small cornea or in eyes with a pannus. Since the haemorrhage is peripheral, it may interfere in laser delivery, especially in hyperopic ablations. Merocel sponges are used to tamponade the bleeding vessels and to constantly wipe the blood during laser delivery. A Gimbel-Chayet sponge may be used as a wick to absorb the blood away from the operative field.

Subconjunctival Haemorrhage

Subconjunctival haemorrhage is a common complication (Fig. 9.5) that occurs due to a rupture of the conjunctival vessels during the application of pressure and suction on to the eyeball. It can be the cause of a great anxiety to the patient and the surgeon must counsel the patients about this complication. The use of a smaller diameter suction plate helps to minimise this complication.

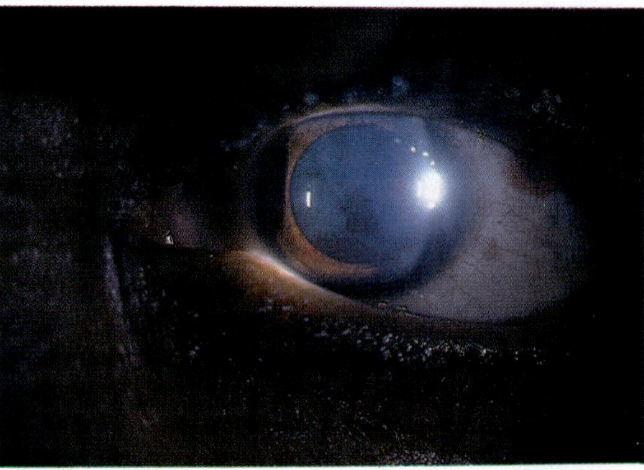

Fig. 9.4: Corneal blood staining due to haemorrhage from inferior limbal vessels

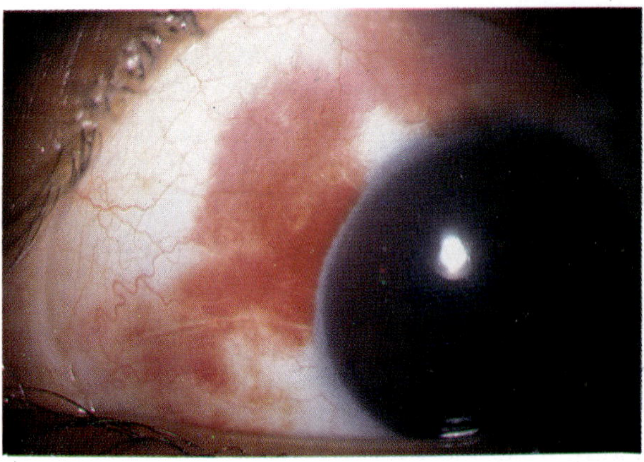

Fig. 9.5: Large subconjunctival haemorrhages after pressure
with the suction ring of the Hansatome

Gimbel reported 32 (3.2 %) intraoperative complications in the first 1000 consecutive myopic LASIK surgeries performed by him using the Chiron Automated Corneal Shaper (ACS) and the NIDEK EC 5000 excimer laser. Micro-keratome-related flap complications were noted in 19 eyes (1.9%). An incomplete pass, thin flap, buttonhole and a free cap were the flap-related problems in his series.

Stulting *et al* reported 27 (2.1%) intraoperative flap-related complications in 1062 eyes which underwent LASIK for myopia, using the ACS and the Summit Omni Med Excimer Laser. The flap complications noted were: free caps, incomplete flaps, buttonholes, thin/thick flaps and bilevelled flaps.

Prevention of Microkeratome-related Complications

The occurrence of most of the microkeratome-related complications (Table 9.1) during the creation of the flap are a result of an inadequate exposure and poor suction or loss of suction during the procedure. A high IOP (> 65 mm Hg) indicates application of proper suction and is essential during the creation of the flap to prevent these complications. It is important for the surgeon to optimise the exposure, to check the assembly of the microkeratome, to perform a full forward and reverse cycle of the microkeratome and to verify the IOP with a tonometer, before proceeding on to use the microkeratome. It is also important to exclude eyes with a very steep or flat cornea, as these eyes are more prone to develop microkeratome-related flap complications.

The modification of the current microkeratome design to allow for a smaller profile, adjustable to fit various orbital anatomies; a suction plate which constantly monitors the IOP; and a direct visualisation of the operative field, will go a long way in decreasing the incidence of intraoperative complications.

Table 9.1: Microkeratome-related complications

Complication	Cause	Management
Corneal perforation	• Improper seating or absence of thickness plate • Corneal thinning	Stop surgery Repair under General anaesthesia
Incomplete flap	• Loss of power • Mechanical obstruction • Suction loss • Debris along track	Stop surgery, reverse microkeratome, release suction, replace flap If cut stops beyond central 6-7 mm, can do laser
Thin flap and buttonhole	• Suboptimal suction • IOP < 65 mm Hg • Debris along track • Buckling of steep cornea • Recycled metal blade	Stop surgery, replace flap Reoperate after 3 months
Free corneal cap	• Incorrect stop mechanism • Very flat cornea • Large cornea	Complete surgery, replace cap

Other Complications

Flap Damage

The flap may be damaged by contact with the blade, forceps or irrigating cannulae. Inadvertent application of the laser to the flap may also be responsible for damage. This complication can be avoided by careful attention to detail and use of a flap protector during the laser ablation to protect the hinge.

Flap Wrinkling

Improper flap positioning, excessive drying of the flap and mechanical stretching of the flap while handling it, can lead to a wrinkled flap. If not managed immediately, it can cause permanent irregular astigmatism and visual disturbances.

The flap should be lifted, profusely irrigated, and smoothened with the help of a spatula or a wet Merocel sponge. The drying time should be 3-4 minutes and the patient should be re-examined on the slit-lamp biomicroscope after 1 to 2 hours.

Flap Dislocation

Decentration or irregularity of the flap may lead to poor adherence and dislocation. If the patient squeezes the eyes while the drapes and the speculum are being removed, it can lead to a shifted flap. The flap should be lifted up, the undersurface and the bed thoroughly cleaned and the flap replaced. Three to four minutes of drying time should be allowed to ensure a good adherence. Sutures may be required in some cases.

Flap loss

Flap loss may occur in cases with a 360° free flap (free cap) or a flap with a fragile hinge. If detected immediately, the flap should be cleaned and replaced with or without suturing. If the flap is irreversably damaged or lost, then the cornea should be left to re-epithelialise, as if a deep photorefractive keratectomy (PRK) has been performed. Surprisingly many of these cases have an acceptable visual outcome although excessive haze may occur in some cases and subsequently a phototherapeutic keratectomy may be required. A penetrating keratoplasty may need to be performed in few of these cases.

Irrigation complications

Excess irrigation may induce oedema of the flap and decrease the adherence of the flap. It may also lead to particulate debris from the conjunctiva coming on to the stromal bed. A suction speculum is useful to prevent this problem.

Interface Debris

The undersurface of the flap and the stromal bed may acquire debris (Fig. 9.6) from the air of the operating room, sponges used to soak fluid, secretions from the conjunctiva, eyelashes and from the various instruments used for flap manipulation. The use of the new plastic disposable microkeratomes also generates a lot of plastic debris. The flap should be lifted, the debris irrigated out and the flap repositioned.

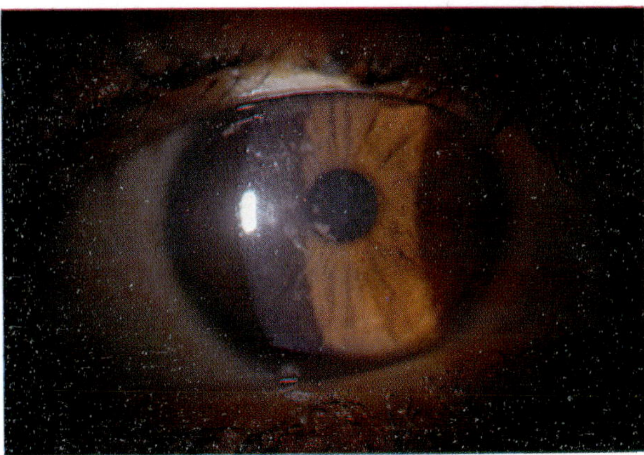

Fig. 9.6: Interface debris

Epithelial Complications

Corneal epithelial abrasions or a loosening of the epithelium may occur due to various intraoperative factors. Excessive anaesthetic drops, improper application of the drape or speculum, patient squeezing while insertion or removal of the microkeratome and damage induced by the corneal marker, are all possible causes of epithelial complications. In such cases the epithelium should be carefully smoothened into position and an eye pad or a bandage contact lens applied. Steroids should be withheld in such eyes.

Laser Complications

Incorrect ablation may occur due to incorrect measurements (regarding the dioptric correction, axis of the cylinder and optic zone) being fed into the computer. Decentration of the laser may occur due to a poor patient fixation or inattention of the surgeon while performing the laser.In addition, interruption of the laser beam may occur due to technical problems in the machine which may be related to the computer, the eye tracker, the optics of the laser and inadequate gas.

POSTOPERATIVE COMPLICATIONS

Complications of LASIK can develop during the postoperative period and some of these complications can be potentially sight threatening.

Flap Detachment

Sometimes the trauma incurred by the patient is so severe that the flap can detach completely from the hinge and may be lost. This occurs especially if the hinge was too small and fragile.

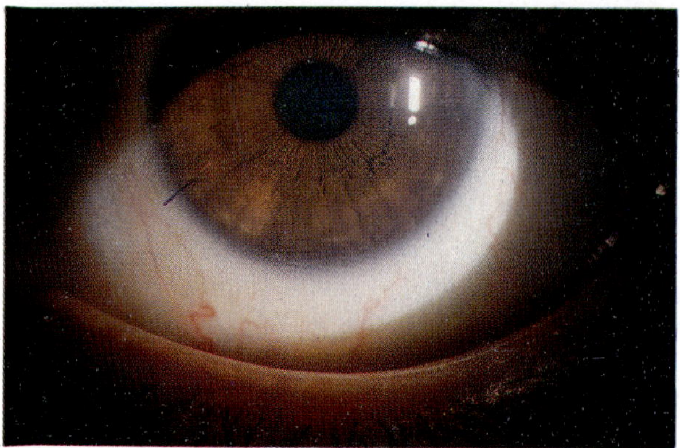

Fig. 9.7: Cotton thread (arrow) under the flap

Management

If the cap can be found, it should be secured to the stromal bed with sutures. If the cap is lost, a lamellar homograft can be considered although often the eye will heal well without it and the operation will effectively become a deep PRK, often with acceptable visual results.

Debris under the Flap

Particulate matter like metallic fragments, dust particles or fibre (Fig. 9.7) can sometimes be found in the interface under the flap. These particles usually come from microkeratome, gloves, sponges, drapes or from other sources.

Management

This debris is usually is of no consequence albeit its occurrence should be prevented by profuse irrigation and cleaning of the interface before the repositioning of the flap during the surgery. However, if considered significant (i.e. if the debris is metallic or at the visual axis) at the first examination, one hour after surgery, or at 24 hours, the flap can be lifted and the bed cleaned and irrigated with copious balanced salt solution (BSS).

Epithelial Ingrowth

This complication (Figs 9.8 and 9.9) is a result of seeding of epithelial cells in the interface or of epithelial cells growing under a slightly raised or folded area of the flap. An epithelial ingrowth may be manifested as an island of epithelial cysts formed by a nest of epithelial cells or a translucent sheet growing from the periphery of the lamellar resection. Epithelial ingrowth is more likely after excessive tissue manipulation and touching of the stromal bed with instruments,

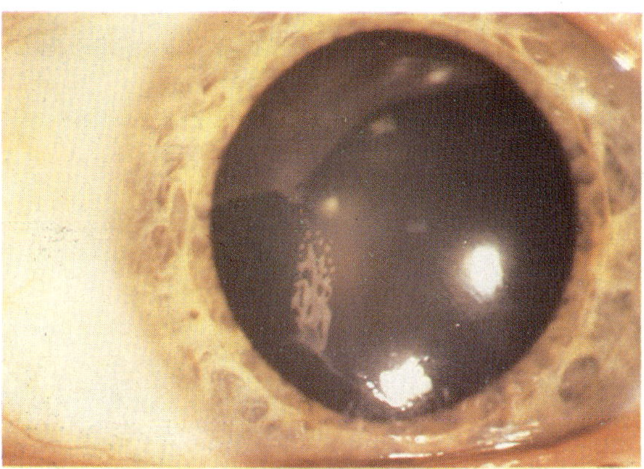

Fig. 9.8: Peripheral epithelial ingrowth

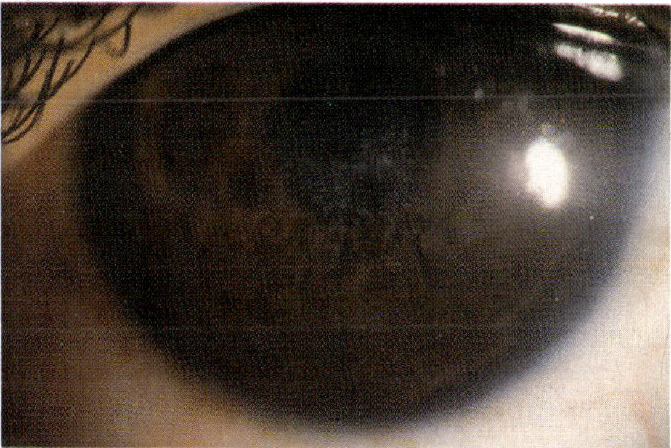

Fig. 9.9: Central epithelial cell proliferation under the flap

that have been in contact with the corneal epithelium. A poorly aligned flap, a flap with an abrasion at its edge, a bottonholed flap or spill over of the ablation at the bed margins can also facilitate the epithelial ingrowth by creating a defect or potential space for the epithelium to grow into. The relifting of the flap for a resurgery also inceases the risk of this complication.

Management

If the visual acuity is compromised or if the ingrowth is progressive, the flap must be lifted and epithelium removed by copious irrigation of the interface with BSS. For long-standing cases, the irrigation is not effective and various techniques have been developed to treat this complication. These include using a spatula or chalazion curette for scooping out the ingrowth, laser ablation of epithelial cells using a photherapeutic keratectomy for a central growth or the

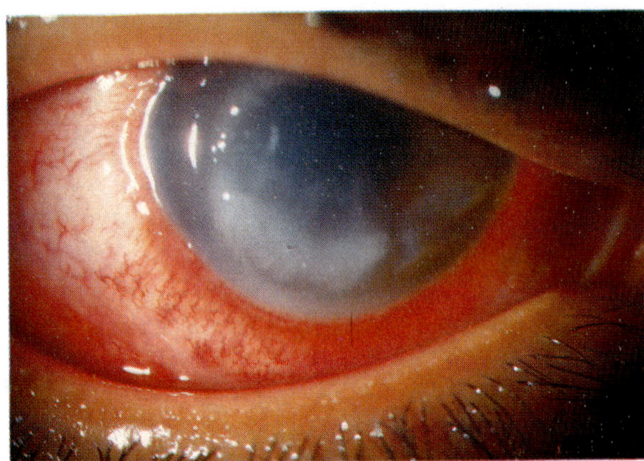

Fig. 9.10: Pneumococcal keratitis after LASIK with melting of the flap

neodymium: yttrium-aluminium-garnet (Nd:YAG) laser for ingrowth in the periphery and incision and squeezing of epithelial cells if the the island of epithelial cells is peripheral. The epithelial cells must be removed from both the stromal bed and underside of the flap. After removal, a bandage contact lens may be used to push the flap against the bed and close the dead space. A delay in treating the epithelial ingrowth may lead to melting of the corneal flap due to the action of various destructive enzymes released from the epithelial cells.

This complication can be avoided by removing any epithelium, tags, debris from the stromal bed prior to repositioning of the flap and approximating any torn epithelium at the edges of the flap.

Infection

Occurrence of infectious keratitis (Fig. 9.10) is a rare complication of LASIK surgery. A breach in the sterility during any step of the surgical procedure or postoperative contamination can lead to this devastating complication.

Management

This complication should be treated as a medical emergency. The flap should be lifted and scrapings of the bed should be sent for microbiological investigations including cultures. Intense antibiotic treatment in the form of a combination fortified therapy with topical 1.3 per cent tobramycin sulphate and 5 per cent cephazolin sodium drops (or hourly fluoroquinolone such as 0.3 per cent ciprofloxacin or ofloxacin) is to be instilled in the diseased eye at 1 hourly intervals, for 36 to 48 hours. Subsequent modifications in the antibiotic therapy are made on the basis of cultures and sensitivity reports and the clinical response.

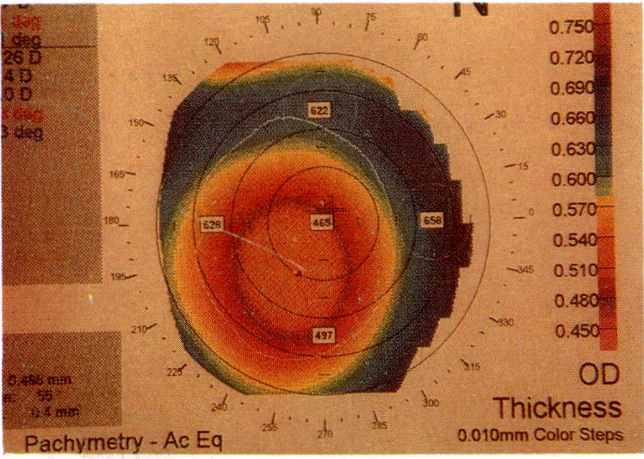

Fig. 9.11: Decentred ablation

Optical Complications

Certain complications can occur during the laser ablation of the tissue and may be related to an uncooperative patient, surgeon's inexperience, wandering fixation or individual tissue response to the excimer laser ablation.

Decentration

Decentration (Fig. 9.11) can be caused by poor centration of the laser beam by the surgeon, poor fixation by the patient, poor centration of suction ring and defective location of the corneal flap. Decentred ablation results in apparent undercorrection and can also lead to the occurrence of irregular astigmatism, loss of best corrected visual acuity (BCVA), symptoms of glare, monocular diplopia and ghosting of images.

Management

Prevention of decentration is the best management of this problem. Most excimer lasers have now incorporated automatic tracking system to help in prevention of decentration. If the patient is undercorrected, then the flap can be lifted and the laser ablation repeated with decentration in the opposite direction, using a wide optic zone. Pallikaris has described a method of moving the centre of decentred ablation by placing arcuate incisions on the opposite side. However, topography-guided LASIK may be the best option.

Central Islands

Like in PRK, central islands have been known to occur following LASIK (Fig. 9.12), particularly if a broad beam laser is used. The exact cause leading to

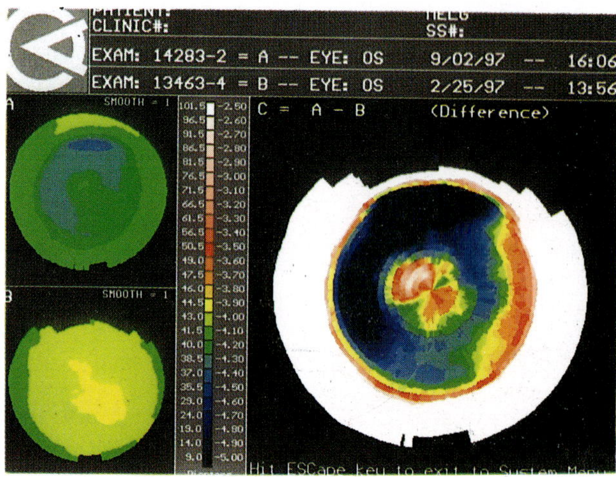

Fig. 9.12: Central island on corneal topography

the occurrence of this complication remains unknown, although most central islands are probably due to epithelial hyperplasia as an inadvertent healing response. Excess moisture in the central stroma subsequent to shock waves of the laser may also be responsible for less central ablation and more peripheral ablation. It can cause symptoms of blurred vision, ghosting of images, monocular diplopia, haloes and an apparent undercorrection. A careful topographic analysis can confirm the presence of these islands.

Management

Certain lasers have incorporated a software for anticentral island pretreatment to prevent the occurrence of this complication. Excessive moisture may be reduced by drying the central stromal bed with sponges during the ablative process. If detected, a conservative approach is used, as in most instances these central islands resolve spontaneously. If a visually significant island occurs or if it does not resolve spontaneously, customised reablation by laser is the recommended approach, adjusting the diameter and amount of ablation to the dimensions of the central island seen on subtraction corneal topography.

Interface Haze

Stromal haze at the interface is rarely seen after LASIK but may occur in some cases of high refractive correction and may be associated with certain amount of regression. It may be due to intrastromal oedema or a cellular response to toxic substances introduced during the surgical procedure.

Management

A course of topical steroids usually reverses this change over a period of 2 to 3 weeks.

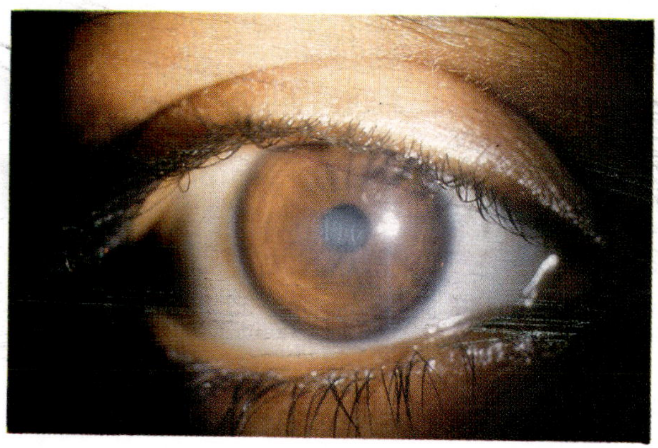

Fig. 9.13: Sands of Sahara syndrome (sterile keratitis)

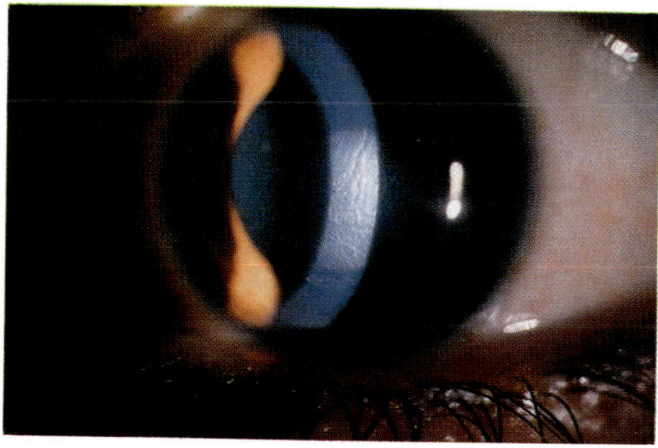

Fig. 9.14: Central disc-shaped lesion due to a sterile keratitis after LASIK

Diffuse Lamellar Keratitis

Diffuse lamellar keratitis is a relatively new syndrome described by Smith and Maloney and is also known as the Sands of Sahara syndrome. It is characterised by the appearance of diffuse, multifocal, non-infectious infiltrates confined to the flap interface (Fig. 9.13) with no anterior or posterior extension and concentrated around surgical debris. There is little or no anterior chamber reaction and the conjunctiva is relatively non-inflamed. Hatsis has classified this syndrome into four grades. Grade I is associated with a localised area (usually superior) of interface infiltration which spreads to involve the entire interface in grade II. Grade III is characterised by a dense, opaque cellular infiltrate with nests of inflammatory aggregates (Fig. 9.14) and flap oedema. The corneal topography is distorted and there is a risk of corneal melting. Grade IV disease is same as grade III but associated with extracorneal signs of lid oedema, conjunctival injection and cells and flare in the anterior chamber. The patients usually present between 2 and 6 days after the surgery with symptoms of pain, photophobia, redness and tearing. This syndrome is probably a toxic or allergic reaction to an unknown inciting agent. Thermal injury, blepharitis, meibomian secretion, chemicals on the blade, rust, betadine, cleaning solution residue, ethylene oxide gas residue, red blood cells, gentian violet, Merocel sponges and oil from the motor of the microkeratome may be the possible causes of this entity. A meticulous cleaning and inspection of all the surgical instruments prior to use in each case may, help in preventing this syndrome.

Management

Although self-limiting, topical steroids (required 1 hourly in the initial phases of the disease) help to expedite the resolution of these infiltrates within a week or two, in grade I and II disease. In grade III and IV diseases, the flap should be lifted and the interface irrigated and brushed with Merocel sponges to eliminate the infiltrate. Antibiotic therapy must be given along with the intense steroid therapy. It is important to distinguish this entity from an infectious keratitis.

Irregular Astigmatism

Irregular astigmatism and subsequent loss of BCVA can be caused by several factors. These include irregular flaps, flap misalignment, epithelial ingrowth, disparity between bed and the posterior surface of the flap, central islands and decentred ablation.

Management

The management of some of these complications causing irregular astigmatism has already been described. The surface irregularities tend to resolve with time. A rigid gas permeable (RGP) contact lens may prove helpful in restoring the vision. Topography-guided LASIK may offer another option. The development of newer microkeratomes, smoother ablations and application of scanning technology have reduced the occurrence of this complication.

Glare and Haloes

Some patients may complain of glare and haloes particularly during the night. This complication is usually seen in patients with a large resting pupillary size or in those who have had higher amplitudes of refractive error corrected. This occurs when the pupil dilates to a size, which is more than the diameter of the optic zone set for the ablation.

Management

These problems usually undergo spontaneous resolution over time and do not require any active management except reassuring the patient. Dilute pilocarpine (one drop of 0.125 – 0.25% pilocarpine in the evening) therapy may need to be given in some patients.

Corneal Ectasia

If a large amount of stromal tissue has been ablated, corneal ectasia can occur. A regression of the myopic refractive error with a progressive steepening of the corneal curvature indicates that ectasia is developing. A tectonic epikeratoplasty, or a penetrating keratoplasty may be the only option available if ectasia develops. It is therefore important to remember that at least 200 μm (preferably 250 μm) of the stromal bed should remain after laser ablation.

Overcorrection, Undercorrection and Regression of the Effect

Overcorrection and undercorrection are common to all refractive surgeries. If an uncomplicated LASIK has been performed, some of these problems are the effect of the individual variation of the healing response. Regression of the ablation effect is more commonly seen after the higher refractive corrections. An under-correction or overcorrection within 1 D may be acceptable to certain patients depending on the type and amplitude of the pre-existing refractive error. An unexpected and a higher amplitude of under or overcorrection than desired may be a result of faulty preoperative refractive assessment, incorrect laser calibration or wrong entry of the refractive data.

The potential mechanisms of regression after LASIK may be : nuclear sclerosis, corneal ectasia, corneal hydration, stromal synthesis and compensatory epithelial hyperplasia.

Management

A laser retreatment can be performed to treat unacceptable under or overcorrec-tions. Retreatment should be performed relatively early in the postoperative period (8–12 weeks) as the flap is still not firmly attached to the bed and can be raised very easily from the bed. A new flap may need to be created if the LASIK retreatment is scheduled after six months, although flaps can still be lifted even a year or more after surgery. The key to relifting a flap is the careful breaking of the epithelial bond. This can be done with the tip of a 25 G needle, a Sinskey hook or a blunt spatula. Before surgery the patient is taken to the slit lamp and the edge of the flap marked with gentian violet on the temporal side. A small area of the temporal epithelium is debrided to expose the corneal flap edge. The spatula is then inserted beneath the flap edge and used to dissect and reflect the flap. A non-toothed forceps may also be used to lift the flap. To avoid epithelial implantation, some surgeons have advocated lifting the flap opposite the hinge and tearing the epithelium as the flap is raised. After the flap has been lifted, the laser ablation is performed in a routine manner.

Complications of LASIK

Preoperative
- Induced by anaesthesia
- Induced by the application of the drape and/or speculum
- Induced by irrigating fluid
- Induced by corneal marking

Intraoperative
- Corneal perforation
- Incomplete microtome pass
- Irregular microtome cut
- Free cap
- Bleeding from limbal vessels
- Subconjunctival haemorrhage
- Damage or loss of flap
- Incorrect replacement of the flap
- Dislocation of the flap
- Poor flap adhesion
- Intraoperative contamination of the surfaces
- Incorrect ablation
- Decentration of the ablation
- Technical laser problems
- Epithelial complications

Postoperative
- Flap detachment/dislocation
- Epithelial ingrowth
- Interface debris
- Irregular astigmatism
- Central islands
- Haze
- Corneal ectasia
- Undercorrection
- Regression
- Overcorrection
- Induced astigmatism.
- Sterile/infectious keratitis
- Glare and haloes

Ten

LASIK in Special Situations

Laser-*in-situ* keratomileusis (LASIK) is a useful modality to treat refractive errors after previously done surgical procedures such as cataract surgery, radial keratotomy (RK), penetrating keratoplasty (PK) and epikeratoplasty. In such cases the eye has already been traumatised by an antecedent surgical procedure and it is difficult to predict the biological behaviour of corneal tissue after a repeat surgery.Since the creation of a lamellar flap demands a high intraocular pressure (> 65 mm Hg), a great mechanical stress is induced on the corneal tissue while performing the cut with a microkeratome. Therefore, although the procedure is effective, special precautions are warranted while doing LASIK in previously operated eyes. An adequate time for wound healing should be allowed to ensure that the integrity of the previous surgical wound is not disturbed. The longer the time interval between the initial surgery and LASIK, the safer it is for the patient and the surgeon.If the cornea has an irregular scarring with contracture that is contributing to the astigmatism, then the lamellar cut produced by the microkeratome may itself modify the magnitude and the axis of the astigmatism. This occurs due to a circumferential release of the tensile forces responsible for toricity of the cornea. Therefore performing the laser ablation based on the preoperative refractive error is not a good option. The treatment may have to be done as two separate procedures, an initial microkeratome cut followed subsequently by the laser ablation after an interval of 6 to 8 weeks.

LASIK after Radial Keratotomy

Radial keratotomy was a popular incisional refractive surgery in the recent past but it was often associated with a residual refractive error. This may be an undercorrection with a myopic error or an overcorrection with a hyperopic error. It is now possible to correct these errors using LASIK. However there are certain important points to remember before attempting LASIK in RK patients (Fig. 10.1):
- Select eyes with a well-performed RK with eight or less incisions
- If the RK surgery was complicated by a micro- or macroperforation, LASIK should not be performed
- If any epithelial plugs are present in the incision, there is an increased risk of epithelial ingrowth after LASIK.

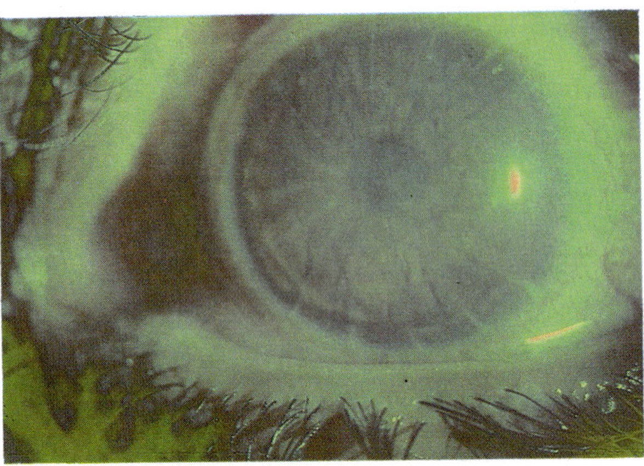

Fig. 10.1: LASIK after radial keratotomy

- The flap dissection should be done very carefully because there is a risk of the old radial incisions coming apart during creation of the flap.
- A 10/0 monofilament suture must be kept standby for an emergency repair of an incision gape.
- One should intend to create a larger and thicker flap (9.5 mm and 180 microns) which is easier to handle.
- There is an increased risk of dehiscence of the old RK incisions when dissection of the LASIK flap is attempted in subsequent enhancement procedures. Therefore a new keratectomy is recommended for a RELASIK procedure, rather than lifting up of the old flap.
- It is best to wait a couple of years before attempting LASIK in RK patients as the cornea is permanently weakened and the risk of an incision gaping, during the creation of the corneal flap always exists.
- It is important to remember that although the results of LASIK are good after RK, the refractive instability and the hyperopic shifts due to the RK incisions may persist.

LASIK after Penetrating Keratoplasty

Laser-*in-situ* keratomileusis (LASIK) after penetrating keratoplasty should be performed atleast 18 months to 2 years after the primary surgery and after all sutures have been removed. One should observe the following precautions before subjecting the graft to LASIK (Fig. 10.2).
- The wound healing should be adequate and it is important to ensure that the wound is well apposed in the entire circumference of the graft.
- No areas of localised thinning or ectasia should be present in the host or the donor cornea.
- Both the anterior and posterior aspects of the graft-host interface should be well apposed and no step should be present.

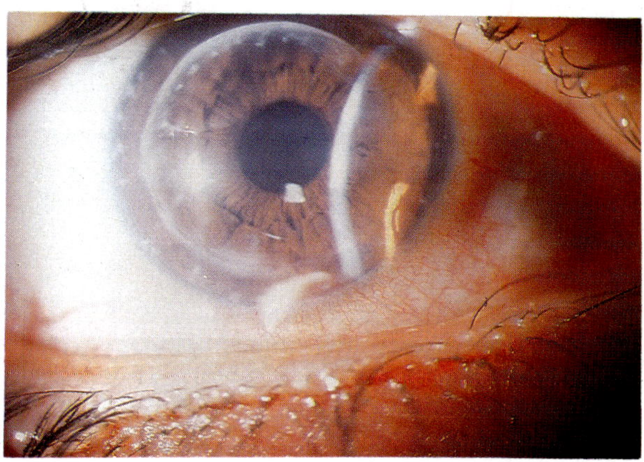

Fig. 10.2: LASIK after penetrating keratoplasty

- LASIK should not be performed if there is a marked decrease in sensation in a herpes keratitis graft. In all other such grafts, acyclovir prophylaxis should be instituted prior to surgery and continued subsequently.
- The patient should not be on a long-term topical steroid therapy.
- Post-LASIK, a 4 to 6 hourly steroid therapy should be instituted and continued for a period of four to six weeks as there is an increased risk of graft rejection.
- If the cornea is steep or there is a high astigmatism, there is an increased risk of the occurrence of a buttonholed flap. A 180 micron depth plate is mandatory in such eyes.

It is advisable to perform an initial cut with the microkeratome to create a lamellar flap without doing any laser treatment. This allows for the tension lines

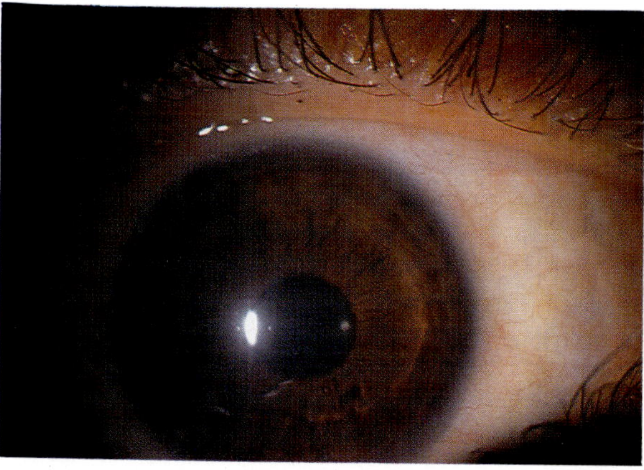

Fig. 10.3: LASIK after epikeratoplasty

to relax, which may itself lead to correction of a significant quantity of astigmatism. The laser can be done after 1 month, or after the refraction has stabilised, at which time the flap created in the initial surgery is lifted up with a spatula and then the stromal ablation is performed. A similar two-staged approach should also be used when LASIK is done in eyes with an epikeratoplasty (Fig. 10.3).

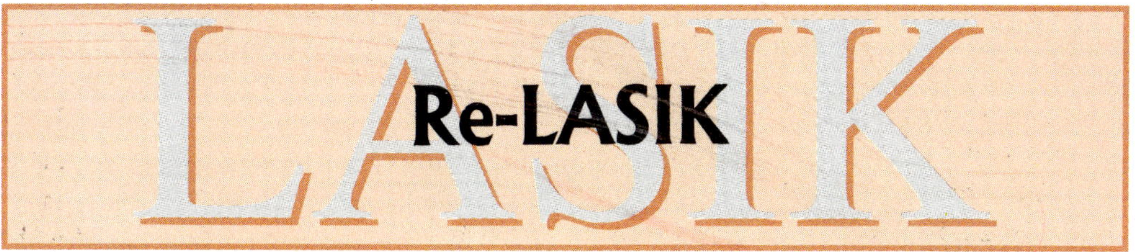

Eleven

Re-LASIK

It is often necessary to do an enhancement for an undercorrection or regression after the first LASIK surgery. The higher the myopia, the higher the rate and degree of regression. Maximal regression usually occurs between 2–4 weeks after the surgery but can be seen up to 6 months after the surgery. The surgeon should develop a personalised nomogram and aim for an overcorrection when treating eyes with high myopia to account for regression. We overcorrect all myopic eyes above 10 dioptres by 10 per cent. Proliferation of keratocytes with a remodulation of the corneal stroma and reactive epithelial hyperplasia may be the two most important causes of regression.

If Re-LASIK is required, it should be done after the postoperative refraction is stable over 4 weeks and can be done after 8 to 12 weeks of the primary surgery. The eye should undergo a complete evaluation including the cycloplegic refraction and the pachymetry. The ground rule of leaving atleast 250 microns of the stroma after laser ablation should be strictly adhered to. If the surgeon had not operated the case himself at the first instance, the details of the flap diameter, thickness and regularity should be sought from the previous surgeon. There are two options for resurgery after LASIK, relifting of the previous flap or making a new flap with a fresh cut with the microkeratome. If the previous flap was irregular, the characteristics of the first cut are not known, more than 6 months have elapsed from the previous surgery or LASIK has been done after a previous incisional surgery, the flap should be recut with the microkeratome. If the previous cut was regular then the flap can be lifted, up to one year (preferable 6 months) after the initial surgery.

Surgical Technique

The eye to be operated is cleaned and draped and topical anaesthetic drops instilled. The first part of the surgery entails identification and marking of the edge of the flap on slit-lamp biomicroscopy as it is often difficult to see the flap edge under the microscope of the laser machine. The edge of the flap can be identified by applying pressure with a blunt instrument (glass rod) at the centre of the cornea or just peripheral to the expected location of the flap. The edge of the flap once identified is marked at its inferotemporal border by gentian violet. A small area of the epithelium over the edge of the flap is denuded and a thin spatula inserted under the flap while applying pressure with the second instrument in the centre or periphery of the cornea. Alternately, a Sinskey hook can be used to break adhesions at the edge of the flap. Once the spatula is inserted under the flap, it should be steered across the cornea to create a lamellar dissection at the edge of the flap. One should avoid inserting the spatula further under the flap as this may implant epithelial cells under the flap. The spatula is then withdrawn and a non-toothed forceps used to peel the flap away from the stromal bed. It is important to ensure that no epithelial tags are inserted on to the stromal surface. The laser ablation is performed as usual, the flap reposited, the stroma irrigated with special emphasis on cleaning the flap along the edges to remove epithelial cells and then the flap adherence verified. Postoperative medications are given as usual and the surgeon should remain on the look out for an epithelial ingrowth.

If more than 6 months have elapsed after the first LASIK surgery, one should recut a new flap. Although this is similar to a routine microkeratome cut, the central cornea is now significantly flattened and this increases the risk of creating a free or thin flap. Therefore, a thicker depth plate should be used in such cases.

Before doing a repeat LASIK surgery for regression, it is important to rule out corneal ectasia as the cause for regression, as this would be an absolute contraindication to Re-LASIK.

Twelve

Results of LASIK

Laser-*in-situ* keratomileusis (LASIK) surgery has been mainly performed in moderate to high myopia. In these conditions LASIK has been found to be more predictable and stable than photorefractive keratectomy (PRK). Also the incidence of postoperative corneal haze was found to be less with LASIK. More recently the results of LASIK surgery for low to moderate myopia have appeared in literature and LASIK seems to be as good as PRK even for low myopia. The recent trend is to perform LASIK for all grades of myopia, and although LASIK has been attempted in myopia of up to 37 dioptres, the results of LASIK indicate that a good visual outcome can only be achieved up to a myopia of 15 dioptres (Table 12.1).

Low Myopia

Although many refractive surgeons do not prefer to choose LASIK surgery for myopia of less than 4D, early results have demonstrated the highest predictability and minimum complications with LASIK surgery in this group of patients.

Table 12.1: Results of LASIK in myopia

Investigator	No. of eyes	Correction (Dioptres)	Follow-up (months)	Postop. VA (% $\geq$ 20/40)	Predictabil. Within $\pm$1D (Percentage)
Buratto	150	-18.96 ± 3.7	12	None	85.3
Fiander	124	-3.75 to -27	$3-11$	81	70
Perez-Santonja	143	-8 to -20	6	46.1	60
Slade	59	-6 to -19	6	66	47.8
Knorz	10	-10 to -14.9	12	77.8	60
Knorz	19	-15 to -29	12	33.3	38.9
Helmy	40	-6.0 to -10	12	75	60
Brint	47	-6.1 to -21	6	66	–
Guell	21	-7.0 to -12	6	71	86
Guell	22	-12 to -18	6	5	41
Gimbel	32	-10 to -15	1	50	–

In a study by Salah, Waring and El-Maghraby, a high predictability of 93 per cent was demonstrated by the group of patients with myopia of 2.0 to 6.0D at a mean follow-up of 5.2 months. Also, an uncorrected visual acuity (UCVA) of 20/40 or better was achieved by 93 per cent patients in this group.

Similar results of LASIK for low myopia have been reported by Bas and Onnis from Argentina. At the final follow-up [range 6 to 25 months], 89 per cent patients of low myopia group [3 to 6D] had achieved a UCVA of 20/40 or better and 30 per cent eyes obtained a visual acuity of 20/20 or better. In the first month, 82 per cent of eyes were within ± 1 D. At the final check-up, the mean spectacle corrected refraction was –0.42 ± 0.98 D.

Using a VISX Star, Doane, Morris and Denning in a one year follow-up study, demonstrated that the results of LASIK surgery are best in low myopia. At the end of one year follow-up, 99 per cent of their patients in the low myopia group achieved a UCVA of 20/40 or better, and 90 per cent of these patients were within ± 0.5 dioptres of intended correction.

In eyes with a spherical equivalent of –1.0 to –6.0D and astigmatism of less than 1D, a UCVA of 20/20 or better was achieved in 94 per cent at the end of 3 months follow-up after LASIK surgery, in a study conducted by Philip McGeorge. In eyes with astigmatism of more than 1D, only 74 per cent could achieve this level of visual acuity.

In a single centre study conducted by Ruiz *et al*, 92 per cent of eyes with low myopia achieved a UCVA of 20/40 or better and 100 per cent of eyes were within ±0.50D, at the end of one year follow-up.

Moderate to High Myopia

Laser-*in-situ* keratomileusis (LASIK) surgery was initially used to treat only moderate to high myopia and the majority of studies reported in the literature have involved only these group of patients. The results of LASIK surgery for moderate and high myopia have not been so good as in low myopes.

Knorz reported the results of a study in which the myopia was divided into 3 categories: –5 to –9.90 D; –10 to –14.9 D; and –15 to –29.0 D. An uncorrected visual acuity of 20/40 or better was obtained in 87.5 per cent in the first category; 77.8 per cent in the second category and 33.3 per cent in the third category. Also, in this group (–15 to –29 D) only 38.9 per cent of the operated eyes were within ± 1D as compared to 60 per cent in group two and 100 per cent in group one. The authors concluded that the accuracy of surgery and the patient satisfaction were sufficiently poor to advise against LASIK in myopia of more than 15 dioptres.

Maldonado-Bas reported that 64.57 per cent of patients with a myopia of –6.25 to –10 D, achieved a UCVA of 20/40 or better; 39.29 per cent of patients with a myopia of –10.25 to –15 D achieved a UCVA of ≥ 20/40; while only 27.5 per cent of patients with a myopia of more than 15 dioptres obtained a UCVA of 20/40 or better.

Waring *et al* published the data for simultaneous LASIK in 378 eyes with myopia ranging from –2 to –22.5 D. The predictability of obtaining a refractive error of ± 1D was 84.5 per cent and 88.9 per cent of eyes achieved a UCVA of more than 20/40.

Hersh *et al* performed LASIK on 115 eyes with a myopia ranging from –6 to –14 D. Fifty five per cent of eyes achieved an UCVA of 20/40 or better.

After LASIK surgery in 150 eyes, none could achieve a visual acuity of 20/40 or better, at the end of one year follow-up, in a study reported by Buratto and colleagues. The mean preoperative refraction was –18.96 ± 3.7D and 85.3 per cent of eyes were within ± 1D after the surgery.

Fiander reported a UCVA of 20/40 or better in 81 per cent of eyes after LASIK surgery, performed to correct myopia ranging from – 3.75 to – 27.0D. The follow-up period ranged from 3 to 11 months. Seventy per cent of eyes were within ± 1D at the end of final follow-up.

Perez-Santonja performed LASIK in 143 eyes with myopia ranging from – 8 to – 20D and at the end of 6 months follow-up, only 46.4 per cent of eyes could achieve a UCVA of 20/40 or better. 1.4 per cent eyes from the study group demonstrated a loss of 2 or more lines of best corrected Snellen acuity.

In a study reported by Slade for moderate to high myopia [–6D to –19D], out of 59 eyes, only 66 per cent of eyes could achieve a visual acuity of 20/40 or better and 47.8 per cent of eyes were within ± 1D.

Brint reported a visual acuity [uncorrected] gain of 20/40 or better in 65.9 per cent of eyes after a 6 month follow-up. The attempted correction ranged between – 6 to – 21.75 D.

Gimbel reported the results of LASIK in his first 1000 consecutive cases in myopia ranging between –1 and –23 dioptres. At the end of 6 months, a follow-up was available in 906 eyes, which had no intraoperative or postoperative complications. Seven hundred and ninety-six (87.8%) of these eyes were within ± 1 dioptre of targeted spherical equivalent and 557 eyes (61.5%) were within ± 0.5 dioptres.

In a study reported by Guell, 71.4 per cent of eyes gained a UCVA of 20/40 or better after LASIK surgery, performed to correct myopia ranging from –7.0D to –12.0D. However, such an achievement was possible in only 45 per cent of eyes having preoperative myopia of more than 12.0D.

At the end of 12 month follow-up, Helmy reported a predictability of ± 1D in 85.7 per cent of eyes that had undergone LASIK for myopia ranging from –6.0D to –10.0D. The same study reported a UCVA of 20/40 or better in 75 per cent of the operated eyes.

Astigmatism

Laser-*in-situ* keratomileusis (LASIK) surgery has been employed by many refractive surgeons to treat astigmatism, either as a component of myopia and hyperopia or existing as an individual entity. However, astigmatic corrections by LASIK have not demonstrated an optimal success.

Ruiz and Slade treated 91 eyes with astigmatism up to 8.00D. At one-year follow-up, the astigmatism was reduced to a level ranging between 1.31 to 0.35D. Uncorrected visual acuity of 20/40 or better was achieved in 94 per cent of eyes at the end of one-year follow-up.

Chayet *et al* used the EC–5000 Nidek excimer laser to correct simple myopic, mixed and simple hyperopic astigmatism with manifest cylinder ranging from 2.00 to 6.50D. At the end of a 3-month follow-up UCVA was 20/40 or better in 85 per cent of eyes. Ninety-five per cent of eyes were within ± 1dioptre of the targeted spherical equivalent.

In study by Salchow, Zirm and Parisi, LASIK was used to correct myopic astigmatism ranging from 0.00 to 3.00D, as a simultaneous procedure while correcting myopia. At the end of 6 months of follow-up, 96.8 per cent of eyes were within ± 1.00D of attempted cylindrical correction and UCVA of 20/40 or better was achieved in 82.5 per cent of eyes.

In a study reported by Condon *et al*, the mean preoperative astigmatism was reduced from –2.20 to –0.53 D after LASIK surgery. However, only 25 per cent of eyes were corrected to within ± 1.00D of the attempted toric correction.

In a study by el Danasoury, LASIK surgery used to correct astigmatism ranging from 0.50 to 3.00 D. A high patient satisfaction was observed and the mean refractive cylinder was reduced from preoperative value of 1.19 to 0.32 D.

In a prospective non-randomised clinical trial, Argento *et al* used LASIK to treat simple hyperopic astigmatism (SHA) [Mean +3.37 D ± 1.62 D], compound hyperopic astigmatism (CHA) [Mean +3.34D ± 1.39 D] and mixed astigmatism (MA) [Mean 3.45 ± 2.15D]. Six months after the procedure, refractive cylinder was reduced to + 0.58 ± 1.22 D in the SHA group, + 0.12 ± 1.23D in the CHA group and – 0.11 ± 1.28 D in the MA group. Uncorrected visual acuities were 20/20 or 20/25 in 66.7 per cent; 60.4 per cent and 76.5 per cent of the groups, respectively.

Hypermetropia

In recent times LASIK surgery is increasingly being used to treat hyperopia (Table 12.2) by many refractive surgeons across the world. Although, the technique has been found to be safe and relatively effective, the unsatisfactory predictabilty remains a major concern when treating hyperopia.

Argento and Cosentino reported good success with LASIK to treat low [2.00D or less], moderate [between 2.00 and 3.00D] and high [more than 3.00D] hyperopia. At the end of 6-month follow-up, 100 per cent of eyes in the low group, 95.3 per cent of eyes in the moderate group and 71 per cent of eyes in the high hyperopia group were within ± 1.00D of emmetropia.

Ditzen *et al* used LASIK to correct hyperopia ranging from 1.00 to 8.00D. In the group with a hyperopia of +1.00D to + 4.00D, the mean spherical equivalent

Table 12.2: Results of LASIK in hyperopia

Investigator	No. of eyes	Range (Diopter)	Follow-up (months)	Postop. VA (% >20/40	Predictabil. (within ± 1D) (Percentage)
Nano	38	2.75–7	12	100	–
Torres	50	2.5–6	9	–	85
Condon	41	2–10	18	80	–
ilino	220	1–5.5	24	88	–
Heryig	50	1–5.5	3	–	100
Zaldivar	576	3.88	–	93	69
Argento	679	<2	6	94.1	100
		2–3		100	95.3
		>3		87.8	71.4
Ditzen	43	1–4	12	86.2	–
		4.25–8		74.6	
Goker	54	4.25–8	19	66.6	75.9
Buzard	14	0.5–1.88	8	93	85

was + 0.33D (range – 0.79 to + 1.45D) at the end of one year of follow-up. The spherical equivalent was + 1.91D (range – 0.08 to + 3.71D) in the group treated for hyperopia ranging from + 4.25 to + 8.00D.

In a study reported by Goker and Kahvecioglu, of 54 eyes treated for hyperopia ranging from +4.25D to +8.00D [mean +6.50 ± 1.33D], 76 per cent of eyes were within ± 1.00D of intended correction at the end of 18 months follow-up. UCVA of 20/40 or better was achieved in 66.66 per cent of eyes.

Ibrahim reported a mean cycloplegic refraction of + 2.25D [range 0 to +3.25D], six months after LASIK surgery undertaken to correct hyperopia ranging from +1.00 to +6.00D, in 58 eyes.

Buzard and Fundingsland used LASIK to treat hyperopia in 14 eyes. The mean preoperative spherical equivalent was + 1.33 D ± 0.50 D [range, + 0.50 D to + 1.88 D]. At the end of mean follow-up of 8 months, the mean spherical equivalent was – 0.15 D ± 0.60 D [range, –1.13D to +1.25D]. Uncorrected visual acuity of 20/40 or better was achieved in 93 per cent of the operated eyes.

These studies demonstrate that although the procedure is safe for correction of hyperopia, its predictability and long-term stability need further improvement. A better ablation profile and effective algorithms need to be developed to increase the efficacy of LASIK, for treatment of hyperopia.

Suggested Reading

1. Arenas-Archila E, Sanchez-Thorin JC, Naranjo JP *et al:* Myopia keratomileusis in situ—a preliminary report. *J Cataract Refract Surg* 1991; 17: 424-35.

2. Argento CJ, Cosentino MJ: Laser-in-situ keratomileusis for hyperopia. *J Cataract Refract Surg* 1998; 24(8): 1050-58.

3. Automated Corneal Shaper™. *Operator's Manual* Rev 1.4. Chiron Vision Corp; March 1994.

4. Barraquer JI: *Chirugia Refractive de la Cornea* (Ist ed) vol-1, Bogota: Instituto Barraquer de America, 1989; 351-52.

5. Barraquer JI: Keratomileusis. *Int Surg* 1967; 48: 103-17.

6. Barraquer JI: Results of myopia keratomileusis. *J Refract Surg* 1987; 3: 98-101.

7. Bas AM, Onnis R: Excimer laser-in-situ keratomileusis for myopia. *J Refract Surg* 1995; 11(3 Suppl): S229-33.

8. Bas M, Onnis R: Results of laser-in-situ keratomileusis for different degrees of myopia. *J Cataract Refract Surg* 1998; 105: 606-11.

9. Brint SF, Ostrick DM, Fisher C *et al:* Six-months results of the multicenter phase I study of excimer laser myopia keratomileusis. *J Cataract Refract Surg* 1994; 20: 610-15.

10. Buratto L, Ferrari M, Rama P: Excimer laser intrastromal keratomileusis. *Am J Ophthalmol* 1992; 113: 291-95.

11. Busard KA, Fundingsland BR: Excimer laser assisted in situ keratomileusis for hyperopia. *J Cataract Refract Surg* 1999; 25(2): 197-204.

12. Carr JD, Stulting RD, Sano Y *et al:* Prospective comparison of single-zone and multizone laser in situ keratomileusis for the correction of low myopia. *Ophthalmology* 1998; 105: 1504-11.

13. Carson CA, Taylor HR for the Melbourne Excimer Laser and Research Group: *Arch Ophthalmol* 1995; 113: 431-36.

14. Casebeer JC, Ruiz LA, Slade G: *Lamellar Refractive Surgery* (Ist ed) Thorofare: SLACK Inc 1996; 14-16.

15. Chayet S, Assil KK, Montes M *et al:* Regression and its mechanisms after laser in situ keratomileusis in moderate and high myopia. *Ophthalmology* 1998; 105: 1194-99.

16. Condon PI, Mulhern M, Fulcher T *et al:* Laser intrastromal keratomileusis for high myopia and myopia astigmatism. *Br J Ophthalmol* 1997; 81: 199-206.

17. Ditzen K, Huschka H, Pieger S: Laser in situ keratomileusis for hyperopia. *J Cataract Refract Surg* 1998; 24(1): 42-47.

18. el Danasoury MA, Waring GO III, el Maghraby A *et al:* Excimer laser in situ keratomileusis to correct compound myopic astigmatism. *J Refract Surg* 1997; 13: 511-20.

19. el Danasoury MA, el Maghraby A, Klyce SD *et al:* Comparison of photorefractive keratectomy with excimer laser in situ keratomileusis in correcting low myopia (from –2.00 to –5.50 diopters) — a randomized study. *Ophthalmology* 1999; 106: 411-20.

20. el Maghraby A, Salah T, Waring GO III *et al:* Randomized bilateral comparison of excimer laser in situ keratomileusis and photorefractive keratectomy for 2.50 to 8.00 diopters of myopia. *Ophthalmology* 1999; 106: 447-57.

21. Enoch JM: Refractive aniseikonia — a source of binocular vision stress and asthenopia (letter to the editor). *J Refract Surg* 1996; 5: 565-66.

22. Fiander DC, Tayfour F: Excimer laser in situ keratomileusis in 124 myopia eyes. *J Refract Surg* 1995; 11(3 Suppl): S234-38.

23. Garty DS, Kerr Muir MG, Marshall J: Photorefractive keratectomy with an argon fluoride excimer laser — a clinical study. *Refract Corneal Surg* 1991; 7: 420-35.

24. Gimbel HV, Basti S, Kaye GB *et al:* Experience during the learning curve of laser in situ keratomileusis. *J Cataract Refract Surg* 1996; 5: 542-50.

25. Gimbel HV, Penno EEA, Westenbrugge JAV *et al:* Incidence and management of intraoperative and early postoperative complications in 1000 consecutive laser in situ keratomileusis cases. *Ophthalmology* 1998; 105: 1839-47.

26. Goker S, Er H, Kahvecioglu C: Laser in situ keratomileusis to correct hyperopia from +4.25 to +8.00 diopters. *J Refract Surg* 1998; 14(1): 26-30.

27. Guell JL, Muller A: Laser in situ keratomileusis (LASIK) for myopia from –7 to –18 diopters. *J Refract Surg* 1996; 12: 222-28.

28. Heitzmann J, Binder PS, Kassar BS *et al:* The correction of high myopia using the excimer laser. *Arch Ophthalmol* 1993; 111(12): 1627-34.

29. Heitzmann J, Binder PS, Kassar BS *et al:* The correction of high myopia using the excimer laser. *Arch Ophthalmol* 1993; 111: 1627-34.

30. Helmy SA, Salah A, Badawy TT *et al:* Photorefractive keratectomy and laser in situ keratomileusis for myopia between 6.00 and 10.00 diopters. *J Refract Surg* 1996; 2: 417-21.

31. Hersh PS, Brint FS, Maloney RK *et al:* Photorefractive keratectomy versus laser in situ keratomileusis for moderate to high myopia — a randomized prospective study. *Ophthalmology* 1998; 105: 1512-22.

32. Ibrahim O: Laser in situ keratomileusis for hyperopia and hyperopic astigmatism. *J Refract Surg* 1998; 14(2 Suppl): S179-82.

33. Kim HM, Jung HR: Laser assisted in situ keratomileusis for high myopia. *Ophthalmic Surg Lasers* 1996; 27(5 Suppl): S508-11.

34. Knorz MC, Liermannn A, Seiberth V *et al:* Laser in situ keratomileusis to correct myopia of -6.00 to -29.00 diopters. *J Refract Surg* 1996; 5: 575-84.

35. Knorz MC, Wiesinger B, Liermann A *et al:* Laser in situ keratomileusis for moderate and high myopia and myopia astigmatism. *Ophthalmology* 1998; 105: 932-40.

36. Kohlhaas M, Lerche RCC, Draeger J *et al:* Keratomileusis mit einem lamellaren mikrokeratom and einem excimer-laser. *Ophthalmology* 1995; 92: 499-502.

37. Kremer FB, Dufek M: Excimer laser in situ keratomileusis. *J Refract Surg* 1995; 11(3 Suppl): S244-47.

38. Kremer I, Blumenthal M: Myopia keratomileusis in situ combined with VISX 20/20 photorefractive keratectomy. *J Cataract Refract Surg* 1995; 21: 508-11.

39. Lattimore MR, Kaupp S, Schallhorn S *et al:* Orbscan pachymetry — implications of repeated measures and diurnal variation analysis. *Ophthalmology* 1999; 106: 977-81.

40. Liu JC, McDonald MB, Varnell R *et al:* Myopic excimer laser photorefractive keratectomy — an analysis of clinical correlations. *Refract Corneal Surg* 1990; 6: 321-28.

41. Maldonado-Bas A, Nano HD: In situ myopia keratomileusis results in 30 eyes at 15 months. *Refract Corneal Surg* 1991; 7: 223-31.

42. Maldonado-Bas A, Onnis R: Excimer laser in situ keratomiluesis for myopia. *J Refract Surg* 1995; 11: 229-33.

43. Marinho A, Pinto MC, Pinto R *et al:* Lasik for high myopia — one year experience. *Ophthalmic Surg Lasers* 1996; 27(5 Suppl): S517-20.

44. Nordan LT, Fallor MK: Myopic keratomileusis — 74 consecutive nonamblyopic cases with one year follow-up. *J Refract Surg* 1986; 2: 124-28.

45. Pallikaris IG, Papatzanaki ME, Siganos DS *et al:* A corneal flap technique for laser in situ keratomileusis — human studies. *Arch Ophthalmol* 1991; 109: 1699-702.

46. Pallikaris IG, Papatzanaki ME, Siganos DS *et al:* Tecnica de colajo corneal para la queratomileusis in situ mediante laser — estudios en humanos. *Arch Ophthalmol* (Esp ed) 1992; 3(3): 127-30.

47. Pallikaris IG, Papatzanaki ME, Stathi EZ *et al:* Laser in situ keratomilusis. *Laser Surg Med* 1990; 10: 463-68.

48. Pallikaris IG, Siganos D: LASIK complications management. In: Talamo JH, Krueger RR (Eds): *The Excimer Manual: A Clinician's Guide to Excimer Laser Surgery* Boston: Little, Brown and company, 1997; 9.

49. Pallikaris IG, Siganos DS (Eds): *LASIK* Thorofare: SLACK Inc, 1996.

50. Pallikaris IG, Siganos DS: Excimer laser in situ keratomileusis and photorefractive keratectomy for correction of high myopia. *J Refract Corneal Surg* 1994; 10(5): 498-510.

51. Pallikaris IG, Siganos DS: Laser in situ keratomileusis to treat myopia — early experience. *J Cataract Refract Surg* 1997; 23(1): 39-49.

52. Perez-Santonja JJ, Bellot J, Claramonte P *et al:* Laser in situ keratomileusis to correct high myopia. *J Cataract Refract Surg* 1997; 23: 372-85.

53. Perez-Santonja JJ, Ayala MJ, Sakla HF *et al:* Retreatment after laser in situ keratomileusis. *Ophthalmology* 1999; 106: 21-28.

54. Ruiz LA, Rowsey JJ: A new refractive surgical approach — in situ hyperopia. *Ophthalmology* 1988; 95(suppl): 145.

55. Salah T, Waring GO III, el Maghraby A *et al:* Excimer laser in situ keratomileusis (LASIK) under a corneal flap for myopia of 2 to 20 diopters. *Trans Am Ophthalmol Soc* 1995; 93: 163-83.

56. Salah T, Waring GO III, el Maghraby A *et al:* Excimer laser in situ keratomileusis under a corneal flap for myopia of 2 to 20 diopters. *Am J Ophthalmol* 1996; 121: 143-55.

57. Seiler T, Holschbach A, Derse M *et al:* Complications of myopic photorefractive keratectomy with the excimer laser. *Ophthalmology* 1994; 101: 153-60.

58. Seiler T, Kahle G, Kriegerowski M: Excimer laser (193 nM) myopic keratomileusis in sighted and blind human eyes. *Refract Corneal Surg* 1990; 6: 165-73.

59. Seiler T, McDonnell PJ: Excimer laser photorefractive keratectomy. *Surv Ophthalmol* 1995; 40(2): 89-118.

60. Seiler T, Wollensak J: Myopic photorefractive keratectomy with the excimer laser — one-year follow-up. *Ophthalmology* 1991; 98: 1156-63.

61. Sher NA, Barak M, Daya S *et al:* Excimer laser photorefractive keratectomy in high myopia. *Arch Ophthalmol* 1992; 110: 935-43.

62. Sher NA, Hardten DR, Fundingsland B *et al:* 193 nM excimer photorefractive keratectomy in high myopia. *Ophthalmology* 1994; 101: 1575-82.

63. Slade SG, Updegraff SA: Complications of automated lamellar keratectomy (comment). *Arch Ophthalmol* 1995; 113(9): 1092-93.

64. Smith JR, Maloney RK: Diffuse lamellar keratitis—a new syndrome in lamellar refractive surgery. *Ophthalmology* 1998; 105: 1721-26.

65. Stulting RD, Carr JD, Thompson KP *et al:* Complications of laser in situ keratomileusis for the correction of myopia. *Ophthalmology* 1999; 106: 13-20.

66. Trokel S,Srinivasan R, Braren B: Excimer laser surgery of the cornea. *Am J Ophthalmol* 1983; 94: 125.

67. Wang Z, Chen J, Yang B: Posterior corneal surface topographic changes after laser in situ keratomileusis are related to residual corneal bed thickness. *Ophthalmology* 1999; 106: 406-10.

68. Waring GO III, Carr JD, Stulting RD *et al:* Prospective randomized comparison of simultaneous and sequential bilateral laser in situ keratomileusis for the correction of myopia. *Ophthalmology* 1999; 106: 732-38.

69. Wilson SE, Klyce SD: Screening for corneal topographic abnormalities before refractive surgery. *Ophthalmology* 1994; 101: 147-52.

70. Wilson SE: Excimer laser (193) myopic keratomileusis—differential stability in lower and higher myopes. *Refract Corneal Surg* 1990; 6: 383-85.

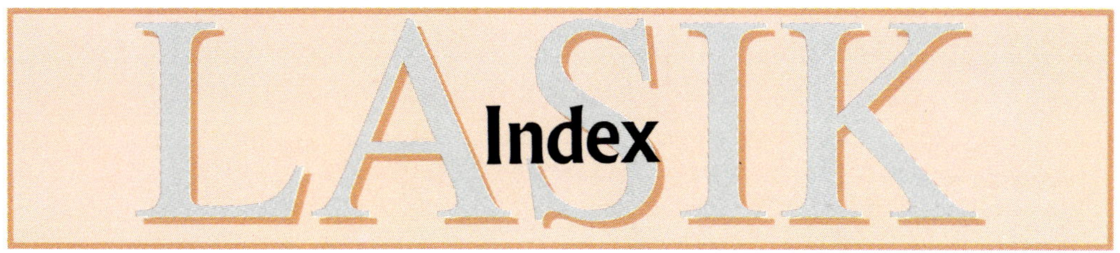

Index

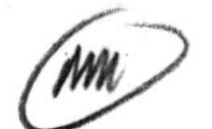